Contested Reproduction

Contested Reproduction

Genetic Technologies, Religion,
and Public Debate

JOHN H. EVANS

THE UNIVERSITY OF CHICAGO PRESS   CHICAGO AND LONDON

JOHN H. EVANS is associate professor of sociology at the University of California, San Diego. He is the author of *Playing God? Human Genetic Engineering and the Rationalization of Public Bioethical Debate,* also published by the University of Chicago Press.

The University of Chicago Press, Chicago 60637
The University of Chicago Press, Ltd., London
© 2010 by The University of Chicago
All rights reserved. Published 2010
Printed in the United States of America

20 19 18 17 16 15 14 13 12 11 10   1 2 3 4 5

ISBN-13: 978-0-226-22265-3 (cloth)
ISBN-10: 0-226-22265-9 (cloth)

Library of Congress Cataloging-in-Publication Data

Evans, John Hyde, 1965–
    Contested reproduction : genetic technologies, religion, and public debate /John H. Evans.
        p. cm.
    Includes bibliographical references and index.
    ISBN-13: 978-0-226-22265-3 (cloth : alk. paper)
    ISBN-13: 978-0-226-22266-0 (pbk. : alk. paper)
    ISBN-10: 0-226-22265-9 (cloth : alk. paper)
    ISBN-10: 0-226-22266-7 (pbk. : alk. paper) 1. Human reproductive technology—Religious aspects. 2. Abortion—Religious aspects. 3. Eugenics—Religious aspects. 4. Human evolution—Religious aspects. I. Title.
    RG133.5E93 2010
    176—dc22
                                                                                2010009049

Contents

Acknowledgments

For general advice on this project I thank Bob Wuthnow, Chris Smith, Paul Lichterman, Jeff Haydu, and Dick Madsen. I thank David H. Smith, Rene Almeling, Mary Blair-Loy, Eric Mitnick, Gladys White, Ronnee Schreiber, Abby Saguy, Amy Binder, and Michael Evans for close readings of particular chapters. For an extremely thorough reading of the entire manuscript, I thank Isaac Martin and the reviewers from the University of Chicago Press. Recruitment of research assistants was facilitated by Peter Conrad, Jay Demerath, Dave Sikkink, Paul Lichterman, Bob Wuthnow, and Chris Smith. This project was designed while conducting a research project on a similar topic with Barbara Bernhardt, David Doukas, Teresa Doksum, Lisa LeRoy, Gail Geller, Kathy Hudson, Debra Mathews, Andrea Kalfoglou, and Nancy Reame. Some of the interview schedule was initially based on the focus group guide developed by this group. Some of the material in chapter 6 has appeared previously.[1]

Special thanks to Chris Smith for repeated conversations about strategies for recruiting congregations, and thanks to Dan Myers of the University of Notre Dame for an endorsement of the project at a critical time. The strongest thanks go to the research assistants who helped me conduct the interviews across the country: Lisa Nunn, Evelyn Range, Devon Smith, David Cook, Rene Almeling, W. David Stevens, Jeff Tatum, and Mark Lacher. Interviews were transcribed by Loretta Sowers and her team. A special thanks to those clergy who not only took that strange call from a professor in California claiming that their congregation had been selected for some kind of study but also willingly gave us access to their membership. Thanks to audiences who gave feedback to chapters of this book: the Department of Sociology at UCLA, the Department of Sociology at University of Pennsylvania, Calvin College, Yale Divinity School, the studies of Christianities Working Group at UCSD, the Genomics Policy and Research Forum at the University of Edinburgh, and the Culture and Social Analysis Workshop at Harvard. Thanks to Doug Mitchell for his usual aplomb in shepherding the manuscript process.

The project was funded by a grant from the Genetics and Public Policy Center, and the Pew Charitable Trusts. Special thanks to Kathy Hudson for support for this project and for her patience with how my new daughter, as well as university and other responsibilities, interfered with my deadlines. The UCSD Department of Sociology was, as always, a congenial place for incubation of ideas at the juncture of culture, religion, and science. The Genomics Policy and Research Forum in Edinburgh provided a hospitable space for further writing. My final thanks go to my wife Ronnee and my daughters Danielle and Karina for making it all worthwhile.

CHAPTER ONE

Introduction

There is a revolution under way in how babies come into being that may change our entire society. Some commentators assume it will "only" create forms of social inequality built into our bodies. For example, a Republican operative, writing about Republican strategies toward societal inequality, mentions that "the trend to inequality will grow even stronger in the years ahead, if new genetic techniques offer those with sufficient resources the possibility of enhancing the intelligence, health, beauty and strength of children in the womb."[1] Some make stronger claims about this revolution, such as that it will change our ideas about what it means to be human and result in the creation of a posthuman species.[2] This is all because new procedures that I will call reproductive genetic technologies (RGTs) allow parents to influence the genetic qualities of their offspring more precisely than through "normal" fertilization by a sperm and an egg after sex. Among the currently possible and potential technologies are genetic carrier screening, fetal testing followed by abortion, preimplantation genetic diagnosis, sex-determining sperm sorting, human genetic engineering, and reproductive cloning.

I will briefly explain these technologies with an example. Imagine a couple who are both carriers of the Tay-Sachs gene, and they want to ensure that their offspring do not have this gene. (Tay-Sachs is a genetic disorder that causes the destruction of a child's central nervous system by the time the child is five years old.) Choosing one of the simplest technologies, genetic carrier screening, the couple could find out whether they are carriers for the Tay-Sachs gene, before deciding to try to have children. If carriers, they could adopt instead of having biologically related children. Alternatively, the woman could become pregnant and then have fetal testing through amniocentesis to determine whether the fetus has the trait and then have an abortion if the fetus is afflicted with the disease.[3] The woman could also use preimplantation genetic diagnosis by creating multiple embryos through in vitro fertilization and then have the embryos tested for the Tay-Sachs gene. Those embryos that express the Tay-Sachs trait would be discarded and one or more that either lack the gene or would only be a carrier would be implanted in her uterus. Another option in the future might be to simply replace the Tay-Sachs gene with a properly functioning gene in the sperm, egg, or early embryo through human genetic engineering, thus removing Tay-Sachs from the family tree forever. Finally, and equally futuristically, the parents could create an embryo that is a genetic clone of someone they know who does not have Tay-Sachs and bring that embryo to term. (For definitions of these technologies and acronyms, see table I.)

The least controversial application of RGTs is to make sure that children do not have deadly childhood diseases like Tay-Sachs. But what about using the technologies to ensure that children do not have a gene that would make them slightly more susceptible to cancer as adults? Or to Alzheimer's disease when they are fifty years old? Or, to have children with blue eyes and blonde hair? Or, perhaps one day, using RGTs to make your children taller or more intelligent? These questions refer to a commonly used spectrum of applications of RGTs, with "health" applications on one end and "enhancements" on the other. A health application is one that ensures that the offspring has a normal state of health and fitness, lacking known diseases, disabilities, and impairments. An enhancement augments or improves the capabilities of the child.[4] Each person will have a different notion of what is "normal," a "disease" or an "enhancement." What often matters in public debate, as well as in this book, is where an individual draws the line between health and enhancements.

Given that the same technologies can be used for both health and enhancement applications, it is easy to see why these technologies provoke controversy. The controversy partly derives from advocates of the extensive use of RGTs. For example, British bioethicist John Harris argues that "Darwinian evolution has taken millions of years to create human beings; the next phase of evolution, a phase I call 'enhancement evolution' could

TABLE 1. **Glossary of Reproductive Genetic Technology (RGT) Terms and Acronyms**

Term	Definition
RGT	A technology that allows parents to control the genetic characteristics of their offspring.
Preimplantation genetic diagnosis (PGD)	A number of embryos are created using in vitro fertilization and allowed to grow to the eight-cell stage. Growth is arrested, and one cell is removed from each embryo and genetically tested.
Human genetic engineering (HGE)	Genes in sperm, egg, or embryo are altered to introduce desirable genetic characteristics into the embryo, which develops into a child.
Reproductive cloning	The nucleus of an embryo is replaced with the nucleus from a cell taken from an adult. The embryo is then induced to continue its development, but is now a genetic copy of the adult. When brought to term, the resulting baby is a genetic copy of the adult.
Sperm sorting	Sperm are divided into XX and XY sperm, and only the sperm that will produce the desired sex of a child are placed in the woman's uterus. If pregnancy occurs, there is a very high probability that the baby will be of the desired sex.
Amniocentesis	A needle is inserted into the uterus of a pregnant woman, and some fluid is removed for testing. The test reveals the genetic qualities of the fetus. If the genetic qualities are undesirable, an abortion is conducted.
In vitro fertilization	A number of eggs are removed from a woman and mixed with sperm. Some of the resulting embryos are placed in the woman's womb to develop into a baby or babies. If only in vitro fertilization is used, nothing is known about the genetic qualities of the embryos except who the parents are.
Health application	An RGT that ensures that the offspring has a normal state of health and fitness, lacking known diseases, disabilities, and impairments.
Enhancement application	An RGT that augments or improves the capabilities of the child.

occur before the end of the century. The result may be the emergence of a new species that will initially live alongside us and eventually may entirely replace humankind." After noting that many of the technologies are in place for the emergence of the posthuman and talking of how humans in the future may use RGTs to genetically design their children to live longer and be resistant to disease, Harris writes that "the end of humanity then is not in itself a concern; making sure that those who replace us are better than we are is a huge and timely concern."[5] Harris argues that it is often ethically obligatory to enhance our children through RGTs to make them less susceptible to disease, and it can be acceptable to make your children

more intelligent.[6] Harris is not some lonely crank, but an influential figure in these debates—influential enough to be a member of the British
government's Human Genetics Commission.[7] Moreover, his advocacy of
evolving ourselves into a "better" species is increasingly shared by others
in these debates.[8]

This controversy will expand as more technologies become available
and the genetic basis of more traits is better understood. Already, many of
the technologies I discuss in this book are in use. For example, preimplantation genetic diagnosis has long been an "off-the-shelf" technology for
traits that most people would consider to be diseases, such as Tay-Sachs.
A reproductive clinic in the United States recently announced that simultaneously testing for fifteen thousand genetic conditions in an embryo
will soon be possible.[9] As knowledge of the human genome improves,
more traits in embryos, not all typically considered to be diseases, will be
identifiable using this technique. For example, blurring the line between
a therapeutic application and an enhancement, scientists in the United
Kingdom have applied for a government license to use preimplantation
genetic diagnosis to screen out embryos that are genetically susceptible to
breast and bowel cancer later in life.[10] Embryos are also being screened by
couples to make sure they will have children without a strong squint, deafness, or dwarfism. Conversely, some couples who are deaf or dwarves want
to use the technology to ensure that their children will be like them and
not "normal."[11] Asian Americans are already using RGTs to insure that
they have a male child in their family, a pattern that is easily detectable
using census data.[12] Finally, in a portent of applications to come, in February 2009 a fertility clinic announced that it would now use preimplantation
genetic diagnosis to produce babies with the desired eye color, hair color,
and complexion.[13]

Even technologies long considered to be in the realm of science fic-
tion now appear to be on the horizon. For example, human genetic engineering has been a futuristic possibility that would allow genes to be
changed not only for the recipient of the genes but also for all his or her
descendants, essentially changing the genetic makeup of the human species. While this has been the holy grail of RGTs for more than fifty years
and was the RGT that first generated intense religious opposition, it has
always faced seemingly insurmountable technological hurdles.[14] However,
in May 2008 scientists passed another hurdle with the creation of the first
genetically engineered human embryo.[15] The technology required for our
"posthuman" future is increasingly available.

Current and Future Debates about RGTs

By and large there are no laws in the United States that specifically regulate RGTs beyond concerns about safety and efficacy.[16] Although there has been little legislation, there has been an extensive debate among philosophers, bioethicists, and similarly situated people about the morality of RGTs and whether RGTs should be regulated. However, there has not yet been much public debate among ordinary citizens like there has been over issues like abortion.

My presumption is that the lack of extensive public debate can be explained by the fact that RGTs are currently used primarily for what are almost universally considered to be diseases, which as we will see has the support of the majority of the public. However, when the first cloned human is born, or the first enhanced human, a debate of greater intensity will begin. Such a public debate is necessary; Should it not be the citizens who collectively decide whether to replace ourselves with a new "improved" species?

At its broadest, this book evaluates what the initial public debate will look like by examining the current views held by the public. Critically, such a debate will emerge in the public sphere, which I define, following Charles Taylor, as "a common space in which the members of society are deemed to meet through a variety of media: print, electronic, and also face-to-face encounters; to discuss matters of common interest; and thus to be able to form a common mind about these."[17] The public sphere is where we as a society debate matters of collective concern, such as whether we should engage in wars in the Middle East, whether we should be tolerant of different sexualities, or whether we should spend the society's money to combat pollution. Scholars often examine the views of participants in the public sphere and how these debates are influenced by powerful institutions such as the media, social movements, and the state. To fully understand how a debate will unfold in the public sphere, one would have to examine all these influences—clearly an impossible task for one book. Instead, I want to shine an analytic light on how the ordinary participants in the public sphere view RGTs.[18] Although these views will eventually be shaped by powerful institutions as a debate emerges, power is not absolute, and the initial views of the public can only be pushed so far in a short period of time. To paraphrase an old adage: One can make a bowl, a plate or even a chair out of a block of clay, but making a functioning car is not possible.

Understanding Religious Opposition to RGTs

The first and most obvious question about a future RGT debate in the public sphere is what the public currently thinks about RGTs. Instead of looking more thinly across the entire public, I decided to focus on the religiously oriented public because I think this more narrow investigation will make the greatest contribution to a healthy debate about RGTs. This is because many of the people who inhabit the powerful institutions in the public sphere that mediate between the public and government officials, such as the media, are fairly uninformed about the religious people of whom surveys show are the most opposed to RGTs.[19] For example, one mediating institution is public bioethical debate, which is a group of primarily academics who deliberate about issues like RGTs.[20] People in the public bioethical debate often talk with the media, teach in universities, serve on government commissions, and make recommendations to government decision-makers while explicitly or implicitly claiming to be representing the view of the public.[21] In recent years bioethicists have split into mainstream and conservative factions, with the mainstream bioethicists associated with the Democratic Party and, most critically, avoiding religious ideas and arguments. The conservative bioethicists have been associated with the Republican Party and are more sympathetic to religious ideas.[22]

Conservative bioethicists who use the religious ideas that animate a good portion of the citizens of this country were dominant during the eight years of the presidency of George W. Bush. With the election of Barack Obama, the mainstream bioethicists are returning to influence. They will be staffing government bioethics commissions and making recommendations about RGTs to government authorities, again by explicitly or implicitly claiming to know how the public that would be governed by these policies would view medical and scientific issues. While it is admirable that mainstream bioethicists want to represent the views of *all* the citizens, since mainstream bioethics debates generally lack religious participants, particularly conservative religious participants, I worry that this debate will not describe accurately the religious citizens' views.

Similarly, scientists are often provided with influential roles in debates about genetic issues. Studies have shown that scientists, particularly the scientists at elite Ph.D. granting institutions who are the most influential in the public sphere, are much less religious than ordinary citizens and very much less likely to be from a conservative religious tradition.[23] Studies of these elite scientists reveal a pervasive ignorance about American religion, typically that all religious persons are fundamentalist Protestants—while confusing the statements of fundamentalist leaders with the views of the ordinary fundamentalists.[24] This book will allow the public to determine whether powerful people like bioethicists and scientists are portraying properly the religious public's views. It is important that bioethicists and scientists get this right, or the legitimacy of their role in the public sphere will be threatened.

I will also focus on people's reasons for opposing RGTs, rather than their reasons for supporting RGTs. This is because the scientists and bioethicists are fairly aware of why people would support these technologies like the scientists and bioethicists tend to do. Why people would oppose RGTs is, in my view, often not portrayed well by bioethicists and scientists.

This study is the first of its kind. There have of course been other studies of RGTs, such as studies of the views of the European and Australian public. But, even in the rare instances that these studies discuss religion, they implicitly highlight that religion is more central to the public sphere in the United States, and that a distinct study is required to make claims about the religious public in the United States.[25]

In the United States, many studies of the public's views of genetic science in general have been conducted, such as the public's view of genetic determinism and genetic research broadly construed.[26] A good number of studies also have examined how populations that have some particular exposure to genetic science by, for example, being a clinician or having a genetic disease, view RGTs.[27] These are not studies of the general public, nor are they focused on religion, so these do not cover the same ground as this book.

A number of survey studies have also evaluated the U.S. public's view of RGTs. Although these sometimes have the religious tradition or religious service attendance rate of the respondent as variables in the models and show that certain religious traditions and higher attendance rates lead to opposition to RGTs, it cannot be determined from these studies *why* this would be so.[28] The few qualitative studies of the public's views of RGTs have used focus groups to look at the public in general and not the religious respondents in particular. These studies may have a religiously oriented focus group in their sample, and religion may become an issue in other focus groups, but they have not focused on religion to the extent I do here.[29]

Therefore, we do not know why religious citizens tend to oppose RGTs. For example, why are evangelicals more likely to be opposed to RGTs than others? The first purpose of this book is then to further our understanding of opposition to RGTs by inductively examining the reasons people give for their opposition to RGTs. I conduct this examination through a nationwide in-depth interview study of members of religious congregations, and a 4,800-respondent nationally representative public opinion poll. These two methods inevitably provide different lenses with which to examine the questions, but by looking through both we can obtain a clearer picture.

Although I am interested in how religious people "think" about RGTs, I am studying how they discuss RGTs, because a person's language about their thoughts, rather than solely their thoughts, influences others in the public sphere. Of course, any theory of why people talk in a particular way must have an assumed psychological model, and my model is discussed below.[30]

Of the many terms used by social scientists to describe the language people use in discussions in the public sphere, I will use the term discourse, which I define as a publicly available system of meaning, expressed through language, that structures how people organize their world, constraining what can be thought and said.[31] A good example of discourses, as well as their effects, are discourses about homosexuality. As little as fifty years ago, the discourse about homosexuality included the idea that homosexuality was a sickness and a source of shame for families. The social effect was severe as some parents disowned their homosexual children and homosexuals faced discrimination in many aspects of their lives. Fifty years later, a different discourse about homosexuality is more available and more often used, in which homosexuality is a natural variation in human behavior. If people use this discourse, the social effects are markedly different. In the 1950s, the new discourse was not publicly available and would never have been conceivable to parents—and thus the contemporary more liberal actions toward gay people also would have been unthinkable. As discourse about homosexuality has been very powerful, discourse about RGTs also will be powerful in debates. A future RGT debate will be very different if most people use a discourse of "playing God," instead of "the eradication of suffering." Although there is much more than discourse that influences debates in the public sphere, discourse is a critical component to study.

In chapters 3–6, I describe what I inductively find to be the oppositional discourses most frequently used by the religiously oriented Americans who also oppose most RGTs. These are the reasons why the religious public is disproportionately opposed to RGTs, and discovering these reasons helps us understand religious-based opposition. The first is what I call the "embryonic life" discourse, that is, "life begins at conception" and to destroy such life is therefore wrong. That the embryonic life discourse is often used is not too surprising given that many RGTs result in embryonic death, and many of the respondents also are opposed to abortion.

The second discourse is "Promethean fatalism," which claims that God has a plan for every person and to interrupt that plan is to usurp God's prerogatives. For example, if God wanted you to have cystic fibrosis, it is not the role of humans to interfere. I also describe subtly different discourses used by other interview respondents that also address the relationship among nature, God, and humanity.

The third discourse I call "individual human dignity and equality," which is that all humans have dignity because they are made in the image of God and therefore deserve to be treated equally. Although we might presume that this is used for opposing all RGTs, in actuality it is only used for some. There is also a related discourse in use among those who are opposed to fewer RGTs and fewer applications of RGTs.

I call the fourth discourse "meaningful suffering," which maintains that suffering is not necessarily to be avoided at all costs, but is instead a learning experience for the one who suffers and for those around him or her. Although scholars have identified a number of other suffering discourses in religious traditions, I find that only this one is used to discuss RGTs, and those who see meaning in suffering are more likely to be opposed to RGTs.[32] By showing how these discourses are actually used, we can see the basis of initial opposition to RGTs in the public sphere.

The commonly used discourses of opposition reveal *how* RGTs are opposed. We can also look for patterns in *which* RGTs are opposed by religious people. The simple answer is that the religious are opposed to more RGTs and applications of RGTs than the nonreligious, but a more subtle answer is to identify the characteristics of different RGTs that tend to fall on either side of the moral divide between approval and disapproval. One generalization we can make from other scholarly studies is that the public makes a moral distinction between health and enhancement applications of RGTs. For example, one study concluded that "the public disapproved of 'designer babies,' but approved of manipulation to correct for disease."[33] At first glance, I find something very similar among my religious respondents. However, I will argue in the conclusion that there are two conceptions among religious respondents about what "health" is that may well be found in the general public.

Will There Be an Effective RGT Debate?

There will be a debate about RGTs in the public sphere in the future, and this book will show the discourses that the religious population will use in that debate. But, will it be an *effective* debate? There are many detailed theories of what constitutes an effective debate in the public sphere, such as those found in the enormous Rawlsian, Habermasian, and deliberative democracy literatures.[34] I want to focus on a feature of an effective debate so basic that it is shared by nearly all theories and is built into the very definition of the public sphere that I am using. Taylor's definition states that, for the public sphere to be effective, people must "discuss" in order to "form a common mind." As another writer defines it, "deliberation . . . lies at the core of democratic citizenship."[35] This deliberation is between people who at least initially disagree. "Both in political theory and empirical work, there is near unanimous agreement that exposure to diverse political views is good for democracy and should be encouraged," write two political scientists [36] So, a minimum condition for an effective debate is that there is discussion about an issue between people who at least initially disagree.

The presumption is that discussion in the public sphere will result in a greater degree of both compromise and consensus on divisive issues. If a group in society feels that issues were not discussed with them, their concerns have not been taken into account, and that their interests were simply overwhelmed by social power, they could become alienated from society and erode the social cohesion necessary for a functioning society. Moreover, on an issue as new as RGTs, deliberation is even more important because it is unlikely that any group has thought through all of the ramifications of the issue. Discussion with people with a different perspective can help clarify one's own perspective. Given the importance of an effective debate, the second purpose of this book then is to help make an effective debate occur by dispelling some illusions about proponents and opponents of RGTs.

While discussion in the public sphere does seem to occur on most issues, thus allowing for the minimal conditions for an effective debate to exist, discussion does not occur for some issues.[37] I have found two reasons in the academic literature why people may not debate RGTs. The first is that, for abortion opponents, opposition to RGTs is part of their opposition to abortion, and the public considers the abortion issue not worth discussing because of a lack of shared discourses. Shared discourses *are* critical for having a conversation. For example, if a secular liberal were to meet a fundamentalist, they might avoid a conversation about gay marriage because they would presume that they have no shared discourses with which to discuss it. Perceiving a conversation about RGTs to be as pointless as a discussion about abortion, the RGT conversation would not occur. The second reason for a lack of debate about RGTs is that the debate may include much religious discourse, which is thought of as the ultimate example of unshared discourse, which would also repel people from a discussion.

Later chapters will show that a future RGT debate *will* largely be part of the abortion issue for abortion opponents. However, I will also show that the merger of the RGT and abortion issues will not have as severe an effect on deliberation as predicted, because, for many people, there *is* a shared language across the abortion divide with which to talk about RGTs. I will also show that the use of religious discourse will not necessarily preclude deliberation. Therefore, we should not be dissuaded from deliberation by initial appearances that the RGT is part of the insoluble abortion debate or that it will be debated in religious terms.

Culture Wars

The concerns about a lack of shared discourse to discuss RGTs are at the core of debates over whether the United States is in a "culture war." The term "culture war" is repeated endlessly in the public sphere by journalists, pundits, and activists as a depiction of debates in the public sphere. Having pundits say that there is a culture war over issues like RGTs can become a self-fulfilling prophecy as participants in the public sphere perceive that there is no point in having discussions with those whom they are told they share no common language. Therefore, it is important to determine whether lack of deliberation—the culture war—is really what we can expect in a debate about RGTs.

Academics have usefully specified what these journalists and activists mean when they say "culture war." A particularly clear articulation is the book appropriately called *Culture Wars* by James Hunter, which claims that debates about moral value issues are not resolvable through discussion, compromise, and consensus—the normal operation of the public sphere—and would instead be resolved through power politics or, at worst, violence.[38] Hunter described the people in the United States as split into two irreconcilable groups defined by having distinct worldviews that could not be compromised, and these worldviews led to opposing conclusions about abortion, homosexuality, and other social issues. According to this view, people are grouped by their conclusions about social issues into two warring camps, with the conclusions about these issues all being "the same" in a very abstract way. By this theory, the people with the different worldviews lacked a common moral language to discuss abortion and other issues; therefore, they found such discussion pointless. Hunter argued that the two worldviews do not divide the religious and the secular, but rather that religious conservatives such as evangelicals and traditionalist Catholics were considered to have one worldview, and religious liberals such as mainline Protestants and reform Jews, as well as secular people, had the other. By this theory, the people whom we interviewed for this project would be fairly evenly split into these two camps.

I and many other scholars have examined Hunter's claims and have concluded that the claim of a general culture war is overstated. For example, I have shown elsewhere that public opinion on social and moral issues is not diverging over time, as one would expect if these were two camps that did not communicate, but is converging, with the important exception of abortion.[39] The claim that there are two monolithic sides of a culture war where issues fall into two camps also has been criticized in various ways.[40] Moreover, most citizens simply do not care about these issues or are in the "mushy middle."[41]

Yet, for all the criticism, we must admit that conflict over abortion and other social issues remains. For example, it can easily be shown that people can, to some degree, be grouped by their *conclusions* on social issues because people who are opposed to abortion do have a moderate tendency to be opposed to gay marriage, extramarital sex, and so on.[42] Hunter provided a general model that was very useful in promoting debate and encouraging research, but we critics of the culture wars thesis have only shown that the extreme version of the thesis is false and have not tried to improve upon it by articulating a moderate version that can account for known cultural conflict.

Due to data limitations, we have tended to focus on people's lack of shared *conclusions* about social issues, which are typically called attitudes, but have not directly investigated claims of a lack of shared *discourses*. But, if we are interested in the efficacy of debates in the public sphere, we should be interested in not only whether people reach different conclusions but also whether people with different conclusions can find a way to talk with each other about why they disagree. For example, I will show that people who are opposed to abortion tend to be opposed to RGTs. This sort of social grouping by attitude is consistent with a situation where people lack a language to discuss issues, but it sidesteps the issue of language itself. We may be in different worlds defined by our attitudes, but can we discuss these attitudes across those worlds? That is what is important for a healthy debate and a healthy public sphere.

So, while the studies of conclusions are important, I want to return to the original claim made by pundits, journalists, activists, and academics and ask whether effective deliberation about a social issue like RGTs is possible in the public sphere. Hunter, building his theory from the classical sociological tradition, observed certain patterns in how people talk about different issues and then predicted that they would not deliberate with those with whom they disagree.[43] I will start with more specific and more recently developed theoretical premises than those of Hunter and then use the data on how people talk about RGTs to describe the possibility of effective deliberation quite differently.

Will Proponents Perceive Discussion with Opponents to be Pointless?

Perceptions of the Fruitlessness of the Abortion Debate

Scholars have not found evidence of a lack of deliberation about most social issues, but have found that people tend to not discuss abortion. Relatedly, while scholars have not found attitude polarization on most social issues, they have shown that the abortion issue has become more polarized over time, suggesting the possibility of ineffective deliberation due to either the perception of, or an actual lack of, shared discourse.[44] Hunter describes this lack of shared moral discourse over abortion as follows:

> It would seem as though there is very little real discussion, debate, or argument taking place. Debate, of course, presupposes that people are talking to each other. A more apt description of Americans engaged in the contemporary

culture war is that they only talk at or past each other. If it is true that antagonists in this cultural struggle operate out of fundamentally different worldviews,
this would seem inevitable. Is it not impossible to speak to someone who does
not share the same moral language? Gesture, maybe; pantomime, possibly. But
that kind of communication that builds on mutual understanding of opposing
and contradictory claims on the world? That would seem impossible.[45]

This is partly the result of specific discourses that logically allow no compromise. Unlike other issues, the abortion debate has been constructed
as, to quote from the title of an influential book, a "clash of absolutes."
It is "an insoluble conflict between two fundamental values: the right of
a fetus to live and the right of a woman to determine her own fate. The
contemporary citizen seeking an ethical solution to the abortion dilemma
must, it seems, navigate like Ulysses between the Scylla of infanticide and
the Charybdis of women's bondage."[46]

The perception of a lack of shared discourse has led some analysts, like
the political theorist I quote below, to advocate abandoning the idea of
shared discourses when discussing the abortion issue. In the normal functioning of the public sphere, people are required to frame their "position
in terms that are acceptable to all participants in the conversation," she
writes. She finds this to be unlikely for the abortion debate, pointing out
that there is not even a shared language to describe what is to be aborted,
with one side saying "unborn child" and the other "fetus." Because of
a lack of common discourses, she advocates an "agonal" deliberation,
where the need for consensus is sidestepped and "participants express
their perspectives in their own terms, albeit within the boundaries of
civility."[47]

Further evidence of the citizens' inability to discuss abortion comes from
a list of projects designed to allow citizens to come to "common ground"
on divisive issues. The abortion issue sticks out as the primary issue that
citizens seem to be unable to discuss without facilitation. For example,
the Network for Life and Choice "uses conflict resolution and therapeutic techniques to engage antagonists across the abortion divide."[48] Finally,
studies in political communication show that individuals who report disagreement in their personal discussion network less often discuss the issues
subject to disagreement. Abortion was the issue that people described as
having the greatest disagreement in their conversational networks and was
also the least likely to be discussed.[49] Unlike most other issues, citizens
avoid discussing abortion due to this lack of shared discourse.

Similarity of Issues and the Fruitlessness of an RGT Debate

Deliberation would then be limited if proponents of RGTs perceived that, for opponents, RGTs are the same as abortion, and thus there is no shared language. Why would RGT proponents perceive that abortion opponents consider abortion and RGTs to be the same? In Hunter's theory, abortion and other issues, like RGTs, are the same—part of the same broader issue—if people use the same discourse to talk about all the issues. This one discourse is very abstract. On this point Hunter is consistent with a number of theories that explain why conclusions about many social issues are correlated, and all these theories hold that the social issues and arguments about them are all part of the same coherent, hierarchical, tightly structured cultural system. Political scientists talk of people's overarching liberal or conservative "ideologies" and social-movement scholars talk about "master frames" linking disparate movements.[50] For example, scholars would say that opposition to abortion and opposition to homosexuality are part of the same ideology.

Similarly, analyzing the debates over abortion, homosexuality, and other issues in the "culture war," Hunter writes that there are (only) two worldviews in American society, the "orthodox" and the "progressive." In the orthodox, moral authority is transcendent; in the progressive, morality is based on human institutions. In my terms, a worldview is a set of interlocking discourses arranged in a hierarchical cone from the one most abstract, general, deeply assumed discourse at the very top (e.g., "moral authority is transcendent"), to more specific discourses that broaden out from the pinnacle (e.g., "life begins at conception"), and to specific conclusions about issues at the bottom (e.g., "abortion is wrong").[51] The higher discourses legitimate or justify the lower.

For example, Hunter writes that "based upon" this uppermost discourse of transcendent moral authority in the orthodox worldview are "certain nonnegotiable moral 'truths.' Among the most relevant for the present purposes are that the world, and all of the life within it, was created by God, and that human life begins at conception and, from that point on, it is sacred."[52] In regards to Hunter's "moral truths," I would call them "discourses about moral truths"; and a number of these would logically fit under a discourse of transcendent moral authority. For Hunter, a person's conclusion about a moral issue (such as whether abortion should be legal) is a matter of "moral logic" that flows from these midlevel discourses.[53] Therefore, while people with an orthodox worldview use different specific discourses to oppose abortion, homosexuality, and other social issues, including RGTs, a master discourse exists that legitimates all of these mid-level discourses (e.g., "there is a transcendent moral authority").

In this model, if you were discussing abortion in the public sphere and asked an abortion opponent why abortion is wrong, he or she might say, "Life begins at conception." If you continued by asking, "Why does life begin at conception?" You would eventually get to the most abstract discourse: "Because there is a transcendent moral authority called God." You would end up with the same final response if you asked about homosexuality or RGTs. This shared highest level discourse is why abortion, homosexuality, RGTs, and other issues are considered in this model to be part of the same, albeit extremely abstract, issue. People on the other side of any of these issues would not want to discuss them with those with whom they disagree because they perceive that ultimately they will lack a shared language with which to have a discussion.

Further Specifying Issue Similarity with Domains

The worldview perspective is not wrong, but rather too abstract to be very useful in determining whether RGT proponents would encounter RGT opponents talking about RGTs and abortion in the same way, and thus signal that opponents consider the issues to be part of the same broader issue. This is because the abstract discourse that links the issues would not actually be uttered in a normal conversation. People who oppose abortion using the "embryonic life discourse" and oppose homosexuality via some discourse like "heterosexuality is unnatural" are not going to use the same discourse for both issues unless pressed to justify their claims. At that point, they would presumably use the same higher-level discourse to legitimate their more specific discourses (e.g., "There is transcendent moral authority"). Then it would not be obvious to potential deliberators that abortion and homosexuality are the same issue for opponents unless a conversation was well under way.[54] Thus, issues will not be perceived as the same if all that links them is an abstract legitimating discourse.

Other sociological theories that are less abstract and focused on how people succeed and fail at forging these discursive links between issues can be used to focus Hunter's theory. These theories do not presume that what Hunter calls "moral logic" will effortlessly lead people to talk about issues the same way, but rather see a greater degree of contingency as people with an interest in making particular discursive linkages succeed or fail at getting people to talk about issues the same way.

The merger of existing issues to form new, broader issues is actually pervasive in the public sphere and has been extensively studied by scholars. These scholars argue that the challenge for promoters of particular issues (like social-movement activists) is that their message gets stale, and gatekeepers in the public sphere (like newspaper editors) become less interested in "old debates." Issue promoters then must continually keep their message fresh. One way to do that is "domain expansion," where "claims-makers offer new definitions for—and thus extend the boundaries of—the phenomena."[55] For example, the more narrow issue of the "battered child" that was based on physical violence was expanded to the broader issue of "child abuse," which also included verbal abuse, essentially merging battering and verbal abuse into one broader issue domain.[56] In another example, in the 1990s organizations devoted to the issue of "abortion rights," such as the National Abortion Rights Action League and the Religious Coalition for Abortion Rights changed their names to de-emphasize the word "abortion" and refer to a broader issue that included abortion while expanding to include new issues. The National Abortion Rights Action League became the National Abortion and Reproductive Rights Action League and the Religious Coalition for Abortion Rights became the Religious Coalition for Reproductive Choice.[57] The issue of "abortion" was expanded to the broader "reproduction," which included abortion and a number of other "reproductive" issues like the availability of birth control. Or, on the pro-life side, activists tried to merge the issue of embryonic stem cell research into the broader pro-life domain, where the pro-life issue had expanded long ago to mean stopping any embryonic or fetal death, in the womb or in a petri dish. Domain expansion is a common enough phenomenon that some scholars consider it to be a part of the natural history of social issues.[58]

Recognizing Domain Expansion

We know that domain expansion has occurred when people use the same discourse to talk about the two previously distinct issues, indicating that they consider them to be part of the same broader issue. For example, a pamphlet promoting the expanded issue of "child abuse" said: "what is child abuse? . . . It's repeated mistreatment or neglect of a child by parent(s) or other guardian resulting in injury or harm."[59] The discourse of "mistreatment and neglect" leading to "injury and harm" is used to discuss the two previous issues of battering and verbal abuse. In our case, we will know that domain expansion for opponents of RGTs is complete, and abortion and RGTs are part of the same broader issue domain, if people use the same discourses to talk about both issues. The use of the same discourses would signal to proponents of RGTs that debating with opponents will be as fruitless as debating abortion, because abortion and RGTs are the same issue.

The existing discourses used to talk about the original issue in a newly formed domain do not disappear—people can still talk about battering and verbal abuse as separate phenomena—but in a new domain a discourse or discourses exists that can be used to talk about the issues as one unified issue. For pro-choice activists, there are still distinct discourses about abortion that do not make sense in conversations about birth control (e.g., "back-alley abortions"), but there is also a unified discourse to talk about the availability of both abortion and birth control (e.g., "reproductive freedom"). Challenging a pro-choice activist's right to abortion, birth control, or in vitro fertilization would probably produce the unified reproductive freedom discourse. For the case at hand, while a specific discourse of opposition to abortion would remain (e.g., embryonic life), the question is whether there are additional discourses that can be used to oppose both abortion and RGTs, creating a unified discourse that would signal that these issues are in the same issue domain and are thus "the same."

Limits of Domain Expansion

Scholars note that definitions of issues are not "infinitely expandable." Expansion then needs to occur at the margins, with issues that can be easily construed as similar, and when the differences are too great, people do not accept that the issues are instances of "the same" broader issue.[60] We can point to failed attempts to make alcoholism a disability covered by the Americans with Disabilities Act and feminists trying to expand the concept of slavery to include housewives.[61] Expansion also failed when the antiabortion group Operation Rescue tried to claim that abortion was part of the same broader issue as homosexuality in order to justify picketing a theme park with gay-friendly policies.[62] Similarly, religious right activists failed to make repeal of the inheritance tax a "family values" issue alongside abortion and homosexuality.[63]

A more ambiguous case is the long running attempt by the Roman Catholic Church to make birth control, abortion, the death penalty, euthanasia, and sometimes other issues like poverty—depending on who is talking—into one big "life" issue domain. In my estimation, this has worked moderately well among only Catholics, and the discursive link connecting all these issues is abstract enough to make the connection tenuous even for Catholics.

Domain expansion is visually represented in the left panel of figure 1, the hypothetical two-dimensional space of issues in the public sphere—in this case for opponents of RGTs who also use the embryonic life discourse. I focus on this group for analysis because they are using the primary uncompromisable discourse in the abortion debate that signals to the other side that deliberation is going to be fruitless. For purposes of parsimonious writing only, from this point forward I will call the people who use this discourse "pro-lifers." Those who do not use this discourse will be called "non–pro-lifers." I recognize that these truncated terms come with baggage, but please remember that by these terms I only mean the users and the non-users of the embryonic life discourse.[64]

At the top of figure 1 is the "opposition to abortion" issue domain, which contains a number of subsidiary issues that are distinctly talked about to at least some degree, such as the following: abortion because the woman does not want to have a baby; abortion because the woman was raped or was the victim of incest; abortion to save the life or health of the woman; and abortion to avoid having a child with defect. Each of these may have a unique discourse that is used in the public sphere, but if the issues are all in the same domain, then there is a shared discourse or discourses for discussing them, as indicated by the discourses printed vertically on the outer edge of the box. In this case, the unified discourse is the embryonic life discourse. The left side of figure 1 is a depiction of the situation where there is no merged issue domain for abortion and RGTs. Below are the new RGTs, without a uniform discourse—they are without a domain.

Existing theories of domain expansion focus on the situation where new issues are absorbed into an existing issue. In the left side of figure 1, this would be where types of RGTs, such as preimplantation genetic diagnosis, are moved into the "opposition to abortion" domain and the language of embryonic life is then used to discuss this technology as well, making preimplantation genetic diagnosis "part of" the abortion issue. As we will see, while this absorption does occur in the case of abortion and many RGTs, we can make domain expansion more subtle by acknowledging that issues can be in more than one domain because there is more than one way to talk about most issues.

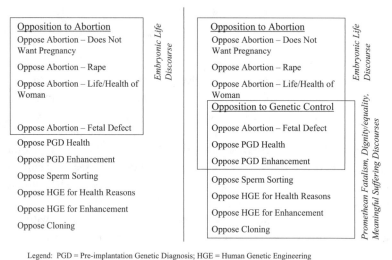

Legend: PGD = Pre-implantation Genetic Diagnosis; HGE = Human Genetic Engineering

FIGURE I. Existing and expanded issue domains for pro-life opponents of reproductive genetic technologies (RGTs).

Scholars of domain expansion say that a successful expansion starts from an issue that can be construed as similar, so the most likely expansion would be from the abortion for fetal defects, because, like RGTs, this involves the characteristics of the embryo/fetus. An expansion is represented on the right side of figure I, where opposition to preimplantation genetic diagnosis is brought into an expanded opposition to abortion domain. However, shared discourses also are used to discuss abortion for fetal defects, preimplantation genetic diagnosis, and the other RGTs in a new issue domain that I will call "opposition to genetic control." The other types of abortion would still be located in their separate but overlapping domain. The reason that these domains are not perfectly overlapping is that the embryonic life discourse that defines the abortion issue domain could not be used to discuss all the RGTs, and the discourses used for reproduction cannot be used for all types of abortion.

If the domain arrangement on the right side of figure I depicts how RGT opponents talk about these issues, then proponents of RGTs would conclude that, for opponents, RGTs are part of a broader domain that includes types of abortion. Other research would then suggest that this would make people perceive that these new issues are "the same" as abortion, enough to avoid conversation about them, like they avoid conversations about abortion. The empirical question, to be examined below, is whether the pro-lifers consider RGTs to be similar enough to types of abortion to discuss them the same way and thus have them in the same domain. Or, are abortion and RGTs considered to be dissimilar, like abortion and the inheritance tax have been for the religious right?

How Domain Expansion Occurs

The scholarly examinations of domain expansion focus on the efforts of social-movement activists, academics, and other people with power in the public sphere to teach the public to link discourses to particular issues.[65] For example, in the expansion of the narrow issue of defending legal abortion to the broader issue domain of "reproductive rights," a discourse was created to talk about more issues than abortion. The pro-choice movement taught this to the public through advertising, direct mail, newsletters, court cases, the media, placards at rallies, and even the names of the organizations themselves.

Something similar is beginning to happen with the pro-life movement, as its leaders are already working to create the combined domain depicted on the right side of figure 1. For example, the social action division of the Southern Baptist Convention, the Ethics and Religious Liberty Commission, produces the "Sanctity of Human Life Fact Sheet" that mostly discusses abortion, but also discusses "designer babies"—a reference to RGTs—and links these issues as one big "sanctity of human life" issue larger than protecting embryos.[66] Similarly, the Secretariat for Pro-life Activities of the United States Conference of Catholic Bishops is publishing texts about RGTs with titles such as "Genetic Enhancement: Custom Kids and Chimeras."[67] They also want RGTs and abortion to become part of a larger issue domain. Having these domains promoted by organizations devoted to the antiabortion cause will further solidify the perception that RGTs are part of the abortion issue and thus not worth discussing.

Domain expansion is complete when the public uses the discourse from the domain to discuss the issue that is being merged in. If, for example, the public already uses the same "child abuse' discourse to discuss both child battering and verbal abuse, then no social movement activism is necessary—domain expansion is already complete. Similarly, if those who use the embryonic life discourse already use the same discourses to oppose abortion for fetal defects and RGTs, then the efforts by activists to expand to create a broader opposition to genetic control domain are unnecessary because the new domain is already complete.[68]

Right-to-life organizations have not yet spent too much effort trying to teach abortion opponents to oppose RGTs using the same discourses. How then could people use the same discourses to talk about abortion and RGTs if they have not been taught to do so by right-to-life organizations or, indeed, if they had never even heard of RGTs? To understand how people talk about issues that are new to them, we can look to cognitive psychology and cognitive sociology theories, where people would use a discourse to discuss an RGT if they have used the discourse to discuss what they consider to be an analogous situation.[69] For example, when many of the respondents interviewed for this project hear about preimplantation genetic diagnosis for the first time, where embryos with undesirable genetic characteristics are discarded, they say that this sounds analogous to the situation of abortion to eliminate a fetus with undesirable genetic characteristics and thus use the discourses they have previously used to discuss abortion for fetal defects. The new situation "fits" with the old, in what cognitive sociologists call analogical or metaphorical thinking; therefore, the same discourses are used for both situations.[70]

How is analogical or metaphorical reasoning determined? It depends on which features of the new and previously discussed issues are salient. An American observer of a room full of people will probably not notice hair lengths, but focus on the sex and race of the people, because those are the more salient distinctions in our society. For abortion and RGTs, we cannot know a priori which features of these issues are salient and thus lend themselves to analogy. (Inferring the salient features will be one task of this book.) In some cases, our a priori intuitions are correct. For example, our common intuition would be that the salient feature in both preimplantation genetic diagnosis and abortion for fetal defects is that "embryos/fetuses are selectively destroyed"; therefore, the situations would be considered analogous. The same discourses then would be used for both, and indeed this is what I found in the interviews. In subsequent chapters, I will present cases where we might think the interviewees would make a seemingly obvious analogy, but actually consider different features of the situation to be salient than originally expected.

For other RGTs, the salient features may be different from those of abortion, because, from the perspective of an opponent of abortion, nobody dies. Rather, what seems salient is that a certain type of person is being brought into existence. It seems unlikely that this situation would be perceived as the same and that they would use the same discourse for this new situation.

The more specific issue domain theory, joined with cognitive sociology, provides a much more precise way of determining whether two issues will be discussed in the same way than can be had in Hunter's worldview theory. The legitimacy of the concern that people will not deliberate about RGTs because they perceive that, as part of the abortion issue, there will be no shared language, rests on an empirical question: Do people consider the situations of abortion for fetal defect and RGTs to be analogous enough to use the same discourses in discussing them?

Expectations That Issue Merger Will Lead to Less Discussion

It is not only sociological theories that predict that merging a new issue with the abortion issue will result in less discussion of the new issue. Political activists also see this dynamic at work. To take but one example on the merger of a different issue with the abortion issue, a January 2009 newspaper article described the strategic debate among Democrats for ending the ban on embryonic stem cell research. The article states that the "Democrats also say they hope to reduce the divisiveness of the debate by framing the stem cell policy as more of a health care issue with the potential to provide new treatments, and less of a fight that spills over into the abortion arena."[71] In my terms, the Democrats want to use a shared discourse of "healthcare" to discuss the issue instead of the abortion discourses, to keep it out of the abortion domain, and to avoid divisive debate.

Similarly, scholars involved with debating the ethics of RGTs see not only the merger of the abortion and RGT issues into one domain as already underway for activists and academics but also the merger as already having a constraining effect on the discussion of RGTs. For example, Parens and Knowles conclude that "the political division that has hampered public policy on reprogenetics [RGTs] is rooted in the vitriolic U.S. debate over abortion. Given the polarizing dynamics of this debate, much of the public policy conversation about embryo research and reproductive policy has consisted of pro-choice and anti-abortion activists shouting past each other." [72]

Others have concluded that the association of any issue with the abortion issue also results in a degree of institutional paralysis in the field of bioethics, one of the mediating institutions in the public sphere where issues concerning medicine and science are debated. For example, a group of analysts, reflecting on a national governmental bioethics commission that was stopped from doing any work because it "crashed on the shoals of abortion politics," wrote that "issues in which abortion is a factor may be issues of which public bioethics deliberation must simply steer clear." This is because the debate elicits "strongly held incompatible views that rational people reach from different moral premises."[73] In other words, people lack shared discourses, so deliberation is pointless.

Of course, academics, activists, and ordinary citizens are quite different in how they approach issues. However, if activists and academics display a condition where issue merger is occurring and that merger constrains conversation, it is plausible that the same condition may be found among ordinary citizens.

Possibilities of Shared Language across the Abortion Divide

The fear for a future debate about RGTs is that abortion opponents will talk of RGTs in the same way as abortion, that the issues are the same for them, suggesting the lack of shared discourses of the abortion debate, and thus discouraging proponents of RGTs from having conversations. However, other social science research would predict that some people on both sides of the abortion debate *do* have a shared language beyond discussions of embryos to build on for discussions of RGTs, mitigating the negative effects of issue merger. To see why, we must again modify the culture wars theoretical perspective.

The worldview perspective presumes a discursive wall between those on the two sides of the abortion debate, where people with different worldviews do not share *any* moral discourses. This is because the topmost discourses in each worldview, and the discursive components that flow from the top, are mutually exclusive, resulting in "opposing and contradictory claims on the world." Hunter asks about deliberation over abortion: "Is it not impossible to speak to someone who does not share the same moral language?"[74] If this is the case, then there will be a community of abortion opponents who are also opposed to RGTs that is distinct from a community of people who are not opposed to abortion who are supportive of RGTs. Each of these communities will have their own moral languages and be unable to understand the other, making discussion and coming to a common mind difficult or impossible.

The worldview assumptions are represented in figure 2. On the left side of the mutually exclusive discourse divide are the people depicted in

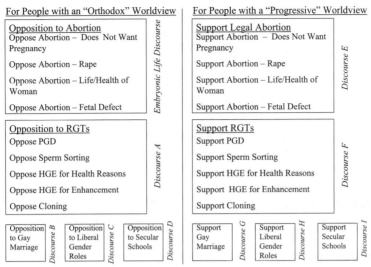

FIGURE 2. Issue domains hypothesized by worldview theory.

figure 1, the opponents of abortion and RGTs whom Hunter would describe as having an orthodox worldview. On the other side are the people who would generally support abortion and RGTs, whom Hunter would describe as having a progressive worldview. The domain of opposition to abortion and its associated discourses are on the orthodox side, and the domain of support of abortion and its associated discourses on the progressive side. Discourses that are logically beneath the orthodox and progressive discourse organize the various domains on the two sides, which would include support and opposition to RGTs. The reason that Hunter was so fearful of a lack of discussion eventually leading to violence was that he saw these issues as all organized in this highly structured manner, with people on both sides of the abortion debate, for example, unable to *also* talk about homosexuality, gender roles, prayer in school, and other issues, like RGTs. As depicted in figure 2, the people with opposing worldviews lack *any* shared discourses to discuss *any* issue. If there is a conclusion that both sides share, such as murder is wrong, they would reach that same conclusion via different discourses.

Again, this is a generalization that should be made more specific. In recent years scholars have begun to question whether worldviews and other high structure descriptions of culture are accurate enough to justify their continued use. For example, studies have shown that at an individual level, cultural systems like worldviews do not actually have a high degree of structure to them, and contrary to the assumptions of the worldview model, people are not consistent in their beliefs, but simultaneously hold vastly different views.[75] If so, then discourses would not be as structured as in figure 2. In light of these critiques, we should follow sociologist Ann Swidler, who has recently called for scholars to "no longer build into our assumptions and our methods the notion that culture is by definition a 'system'" (e.g., like a worldview) and instead find a way to describe the intermediate levels of structure that we see.[76] Issue domains are this sort of intermediate-level structure.

We can use other scholars' research to try to stake out an interme-diate position in evaluating whether there is shared discourse across the abortion divide. One logical extreme would be that the very premise of a discursive divide is wrong and people on opposing sides of the abortion debate actually use the exact same moral languages to discuss abortion. If so, then there would be no concern of an ineffective public debate due to a lack of shared moral languages. However, empirical research suggests that people on opposing sides of the abortion debate do not use the same moral discourses to discuss abortion. Beyond the obvious difference in how they talk about embryos and fetuses, Michelle Dillon, summarizing qualitative studies of abortion activists, writes that activists on the two sides "express very different understandings of sexual morality, and dis-agree as to whether motherhood and gender roles are natural or socially constructed."[77]

We can also a priori eliminate the other extreme claim that the ab-solute mutual exclusivity of moral languages between antiabortion and pro-choice advocates means that they do not use a moral discourse that the other side would use for *any* issue, as is implied in figure 2. This is obviously incorrect, as nearly everyone in the United States shares some moral languages (e.g., "It is better to do good than harm"). The perfect organization of all issues and discourses into two sides organized by the abortion debate is one of the overstatements in the culture wars thesis that has been criticized by many scholars.

Between the two logical extremes of an impregnable discursive divide and a lack of any divide, we need a description of the somewhat porous divide that clearly exists. For example, on the abortion issue, Dillon con-cludes that "both sides share basic value commitments as exemplified by their affirmation of motherhood, concern with women's social status, and sensitivity to the moral and practical implications of both pregnancy and abortion."[78] That is, the people on both sides of the abortion debate use different discourses to discuss abortion, but used the same discourses on issues that were somewhat conceptually distant from the abortion issue.

For shared discourses to assist in conversation, they need to be drawn from issues proximate to the issue over which there is a disagreement. If Dillon were to have concluded that women on both sides of the abortion debate share a discourse about global warming, this would be less relevant, because it is hard to build a conversation about abortion from global warming. Therefore, there will be less chance of diminished deliberation, and thus an ineffective debate, if there is a shared discourse across the abortion divide on a very similar issue to the one that is the subject of disagreement.[79] If people on the two sides disagree about preimplantation genetic diagnosis for cystic fibrosis and use different languages to state this opposition, do they have a shared discourse on the related issue of preimplantation genetic diagnosis for sex selection? There should be less concern over the merger of the abortion and RGT issues leading to perceptions of a lack of shared discourses with which to deliberate if at least some people on both sides of the abortion debate actually share discourses that could be used as the basis of a conversation about RGTs. We can look for these shared discourses by looking in great detail at how people discuss these issues.

Preview of Findings and Outline of Book

I recognize that I have used many terms in this introduction. Moreover, talk of culture wars, opposing worldviews, and irreconcilable debates are so dominant in the media, as well as in the social sciences, that it may be hard to understand a contrasting theoretical perspective. Therefore, I will preview the findings so the substantive chapters are easier to follow. In chapter 2, I provide a historical background of RGTs. Tracing these technologies back to the eugenics movements of the nineteenth century, I discuss the reaction of religious communities to these technologies as they developed and complete the chapter by providing basic survey results on the level of opposition to different RGTs by members of different religious traditions.

Figure 3 summarizes the findings in chapters 3–6, where each of the four most prevalent discourses of the opponents is examined. On the left side are the pro-lifers and on the right side the non–pro-lifers, which

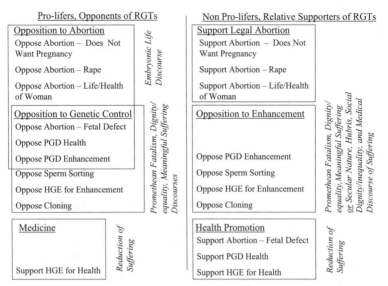

Legend: PGD = Pre-implantation Genetic Diagnosis; HGE = Human Genetic Engineering; RGT = Reproductive Genetic Technology

FIGURE 3. Actual issue domains for abortion and reproductive genetic technologies (RGTs).

represents not only the one known culture war divide but also one of the irreconcilable positions in the abortion debate that leads to a lack of discussion. If I can find the grounds for discussion across this divide, one can expect to find it across weaker divides. Those on the left are also the stronger opponents of RGTs, and on the right the (relative) proponents of RGTs. Those on the right are relative and not absolute proponents because almost nobody in the United States is in favor of enhancements like reproductive cloning and producing heritable increases in intelligence. The fact that the opponents of RGTs also tend to be the opponents of abortion, and that the (relative) proponents of RGTs tend to be supporters of legal abortion, shows that there is indeed some structure to the *conclusions* in the public sphere. The two sides reach distinct conclusions, but do they use distinct discourses to do so?

The opposition to abortion domain from the right panel of figure 1 is replicated on the left side of figure 3. The question in chapter 3 is whether pro-lifers only use the embryonic life discourse to oppose abortion. Visually, this would be represented by moving the "opposition to abortion" domain box so it does not overlap with the "opposition to genetic control" domain box, because there would be no shared discourses. I find that some of those who use the embryonic life discourse to oppose abortion do *only* use this discourse, with the predictable effect that they see RGTs that do not result in embryonic death to be entirely different issues. If this were the dominant view among those who use the embryonic life discourse, then there would be no concern about the viability of future discussions, because the RGT and the abortion issues would be perceived to be un-related. However, I also show that such people are relatively rare, and that the dominant pattern is the merged issues depicted on the left side of figure 3.[80]

In chapters 4–6, I focus on the other three discourses used by the stron-gest opponents of RGTs: Promethean fatalism, individual dignity/equality, and meaningful suffering. In each chapter I discuss the discourse in detail and show variations in use by the religious community. The presentation of which RGTs are discussed with which discourse follows the flow of the typical in-depth interview. The interviews start with discussing abortion for a fetal defect, which I represent by asking about the morality of abort-ing a fetus that has cystic fibrosis. (Cystic fibrosis is a genetically inherited condition where mucus clogs the lungs and leads to life-threatening lung infections. Whereas in the fifties most children with cystic fibrosis died be-fore they started school, today many people with cystic fibrosis can expect to live into their thirties or forties.)[81]

Social science research and theories that consider the embryonic life discourse to be the only discourse used by pro-lifers to oppose abortion leads to the conclusion that there is no shared discourse across the abor-tion divide. However, I find that the pro-lifers *also* tend to use the Pro-methean fatalist, individual dignity/equality, and meaningful suffering discourses to discuss abortion for cystic fibrosis. This is indicated in the left side of figure 3 by this issue's simultaneous location in the overlapping domain called "opposition to genetic control," defined by the three latter discourses, which are printed vertically on the side of the box represent-ing the domain. Although you might think that logically all that people would use to oppose abortion is embryonic life discourse, it is clear that for most of this group abortion for cystic fibrosis is similar to a more varied set of situations than to only killing persons. For example, the use of the meaningful suffering discourse in this situation means that not having an abortion and therefore having a child with cystic fibrosis is similar to other situations of meaningful suffering for the respondents. For our purposes, what is important is that through a more detailed analysis of the discourse of opposition to abortion for cystic fibrosis, we see that these four dis-courses are used.

Respondents were then asked about preimplantation genetic diagnosis for cystic fibrosis; this situation only differs from abortion for cystic fibrosis by the age of the embryo/fetus and its physical location in a petri dish instead of a uterus. For most pro-lifers, the age of the embryo/fetus and its physical location do not seem to be salient features of the new situation, so it is not surprising that these situations are considered to be analogous and the same four discourses are used. This is indicated on the left side of figure 3 by preimplantation genetic diagnosis applications being in the same two domains as abortion for cystic fibrosis. Preimplantation genetic diagnosis applications are "the same" as abortion for the pro-lifers.

However, when a new situation is described in the interview where embryonic life no longer "fits," such as using an enhancement like sperm sorting to guarantee the birth of a boy (which offers no threat to embryos), they continue to use the other three discourses they used for the abortion discussion without the embryonic life discourse. Opposition to these new issues is located in the "opposition to genetic control domain" due to reliance on the three latter discourses. This means that observers who worry about the merger of these issues are correct. Pro-lifers do see them as the same.

However, while theories predicting merger are right, the conclusion that this then means there will be no shared discourses across the abortion divide is wrong. Examining the right side of figure 3, as you would expect, the non–pro-lifers generally do not oppose abortion for cystic fibrosis, nor do they oppose what they consider "health" applications of RGTs, instead using a discourse of the reduction of suffering, which places these RGT applications in a distinct domain I call "health promotion."

These (relative) supporters of RGTs nonetheless typically reach the same conclusions about the RGTs that produce enhancements as do those on the other side of the abortion divide. These people then have their own domain for these issues that I call "opposition to genetic enhancement." Many of these respondents use different discourses than those on the other side of the debate to reach these conclusions. We will examine these discourses in each chapter (and they are the second set listed vertically next to the "opposition to genetic enhancement" domain on the right of fig. 3). Importantly for future deliberation, these people *do* live in a distinct discursive world, sharing almost no discourses about RGTs with those on the other side of the abortion issue.

But, critically, for others on the non–pro-lifer side, the same discourses are used to state their opposition to enhancements as are used on the other side of the supposed discursive divide. Instead of Hunter's worldview perspective portrayed in figure 2 where the domains and their discourses are all neatly sorted into two mutually exclusive sides, the reality is that a divide on one issue like abortion does not automatically create a discursive divide in another, and many of the people on both sides of the abortion debate agree on some issues using the same discourse. Moreover, this means that strong opponents and many of the (relative) proponents of RGTs have a shared language for an issue they agree on like sperm sorting, an issue that is extremely similar to issues that they disagree on, like RGTs for health reasons, and for the abortion issue itself. This suggests that common discursive ground for issues where disagreement remains may not be too elusive and that deliberation may well be possible.

There remains the seemingly peculiar case of human genetic engineering for cystic fibrosis. As described to the respondents during the interview, this involves changing the genes in an embryo to remove cystic fibrosis from the resulting person and that person's descendants. This issue is seemingly similar to sperm sorting in that we portrayed it as not resulting in embryonic destruction. Yet, unlike the discussion of sperm sorting, abortion opponents tend to not use the discourses from the abortion discussion to oppose this RGT and therefore do not see it as the same situation as abortion for cystic fibrosis. In fact, as I will elaborate in later chapters, they are often supportive of human genetic engineering for cystic fibrosis. Human genetic engineering for cystic fibrosis is then, for people on both sides of the abortion divide, in distinct domains defined by the discourse of the reduction of suffering. There is then this one more nearly universally shared discourse across the abortion divide, on this one issue, on which a conversation could be built.

The specific conclusions about this particular RGT suggest the usefulness of my more specific theory of issue similarity. While more general theories would lump all RGTs together, my analysis shows that for abortion opponents, human genetic engineering for health reasons is an utterly unrelated issue to not only abortion but also to the other RGTs. Discussion about this issue can proceed independently of the limitations of these other debates.

Finally, in chapter 7, I separately evaluate the second reason that people may not want to discuss RGTs—that people will be using religious language. I conclude that if there is going to be a lack of debate about RGTs in the future, it is not going to be because the debate has religious content. Respondents want to talk with each other religiously and, inverting the common concern about religion leading to misunderstanding, feel that speaking religiously *increases* our understanding of each other's arguments. In the conclusion, I summarize these findings, point out limitations of this study, and make some cautious predictions about the future RGT debate.

Which Religious People?

On the one hand, it would be interesting to see how members of each religious tradition in the United States discuss reproductive genetics. There are Hindus, Muslims, Pagans, Zoroastrians, and many other groups in the United States, all of which will be participating in a future debate. This would be impractical. Like almost all research that tries to make claims about the general public, smaller religious traditions cannot be examined, and much of the variation within the large traditions has to be glossed over. My concern with the public debate over RGTs also makes examining the diversity of religion in the United States less important than representing the religious traditions that are likely to have an influence on public debates. Therefore, I examine Roman Catholics, conservative Protestants (evangelicals and fundamentalists), mainline and liberal Protestants, Jews, and "seculars." The first three are the largest traditions in the United States and have long been involved with debates in the public sphere.

The decision to include Jews is less obvious, given that they are a very small religious minority, with about as many members as religious traditions that I am excluding such as Islam. The primary reason for this is that, despite the smaller number of Jews in the United States, there are many leaders of Jewish organizations that advocate for policies concerning genetics. The same cannot be said for the other religious minorities. Jewish groups are fairly attentive to issues of genetics for two reasons. First, while there may be genetic traits associated with members of other religious minority groups, Jews are very aware of genetic traits found disproportionately among themselves, such as Tay-Sachs disease. Second, the sad history of eugenics took place at the expense of the Jewish people, with the Nazis claiming that genetically inferior "races," such as the Jews, had to be killed in the name of genetic purity. In sum, despite their smaller number in the United States, Jews will be involved in any public debate in genetics and thus are important to study.

In a study of religious groups, including "seculars" may seem to be an odd decision. I do not want to enter debates about whether secularism is a type of functional religion, but rather I study "seculars" for the pragmatic reason that it is methodologically difficult to isolate discourses that are particularly religious without having a nonreligious discourse with which to compare. Seculars as I define them do not even have to be agnostic—they could believe in God—but must be disconnected from the discourse of any religious tradition. For example, by my working definition, they could not attend religious services. I treat the seculars like the religious groups in the analysis, and it is informative to see where they fit on the spectrum with the other groups.

To see how I defined each of these religious groups during the research, refer to the Methodological Appendix. However, a brief description of these different groups is useful. In the United States, the vast majority of Jews are members of the reform and conservative movements. Both define themselves in relation to the orthodox movement, which aspires to practice Judaism as it was practiced hundreds of years ago. The reform movement was an earlier innovation than conservatism, and it was an attempt to make Judaism more relevant by removing orthodox religious restrictions that they perceived as not fitting with the modern world. So, especially early in the movement, Reform Jews did not maintain the kosher dietary restrictions or wear the distinctive clothing that Jews have traditionally worn. The conservative movement is located between reform and orthodoxy in all these characteristics. A much smaller movement, Reconstructionism, is an offshoot of the conservative movement and is ritualistically similar to the conservative movement but socially and theologically much more liberal.

Catholicism is not monolithic; rather, various factions are located within this tradition, albeit sorted to some extent by congregation. For simplicity, we can say that there are traditionalists, moderates, and liberals. Traditionalists follow more of the rules and teachings of the church and are more respectful of papal authority. Liberals are at the opposite end of the spectrum, being more skeptical of the authority of the leadership and believing more in the freedom of individual Catholics to set their own minds on matters such as RGTs. The label "moderate" is for people who do not want to embrace either of these extremes.

There is a good degree of academic consensus about the definitions described immediately above. There is less consensus about categorizing different types of Protestants. Mainline or liberal Protestants are the theological descendants of not only the reformation but also the modernists of the 1930s.[82] Liberal in theology, mainline Protestants have never dominated numerically the religious landscape, although they did dominate the social and political landscape of the United States for many years and continue to have influence disproportionate to their numbers.[83] Although mainline Protestants can be found in most Protestant denominations, usually they are thought of as clustering within a number of historically mainline denominations. The six largest mainline denominations are the United Methodist Church, the Episcopal Church, the Presbyterian Church (USA), the United Church of Christ, the Evangelical Lutheran Church in America, and the American Baptist Churches.[84] Regarding some of the usual ways that Protestants theologically distinguish themselves, mainline Protestants are generally not biblical literalists and do not believe that the Kingdom of God will arrive in a violent end-times scenario of Armageddon and rapture. They are more likely to believe that we humans are to create the Kingdom of God on earth through our benevolent actions, rather than via the violent second coming of the Christ.

Evangelical and fundamentalist Protestants became more widely discussed in the 1980s with the rise of the religious right, and, more recently, because former President George W. Bush is a member of the evangelical tradition. I will also use the term "conservative Protestant" to describe evangelicals and fundamentalists using the same term, and this is the largest religious tradition in the United States. When people who are unfamiliar with the details of American religion encounter a conservative Protestant, they tend to call them a "fundamentalist," but, in actuality, fundamentalists are a very small component of the conservative Protestant group, with evangelicals being the far larger group.[85] As a generalization, we can say that evangelicals are more liberal than fundamentalists, although obviously liberalism is a relative term. Fundamentalists believe in what they consider to be "the fundamentals" of the Christian faith, including biblical inerrancy, the Virgin birth, and the bodily resurrection of Jesus. They are more socially separatist than other conservative Protestants. Fundamentalists typically have socially conservative perspectives on most social issues.

Evangelicalism is itself a broad term. Underneath this category are Pentecostals (people who speak in tongues and perhaps engage in faith healing), what I will call "traditional evangelicals," such as Southern Baptists and Nazarenes, as well as "nontraditional evangelicals" who belong to congregations where informality in worship style and dress are common.[86] Evangelicalism is theologically located between fundamentalism and liberal Protestantism. Indeed, it was consciously invented to hold that role.[87] While evangelicals can be found in most Protestant denominations, they are concentrated in some more than others. For example, odds are that a Southern Baptist will be either an evangelical or a fundamentalist, and not a liberal Protestant. The same could be said of the Christian and Missionary Alliance, the Presbyterian Church in America, the Christian Reform Church, the Assemblies of God, and many others.[88]

Methods

There are two sources of data in this book: interviews with 145 members of religious congregations and 35 secular people across the United States, as well as a nationally representative public opinion poll.[89] The respondents to the nationally representative survey were selected by using standard social science techniques. For the in-depth interviewees, the number of respondents in each religious category roughly represents the percentage of members of religious congregations in the United States who are in that category. In addition to the broad categories mentioned above (e.g., evangelicalism), I tried to make sure that known variation within each of these categories was represented. So, for example, among the conservative Protestant interviewees, I made sure to have appropriate numbers of Pentecostals, fundamentalists, traditional evangelicals, and nontraditional evangelicals. Given that there are more evangelicals in the churchgoing population of the United States than there are mainline Protestants, there are more evangelicals in my interview pool. For more methodological details, please refer to the methodological appendix.

Notes to Readers outside the Social Sciences

This book is squarely in the sociological tradition, using sociological methods, theories, and forms of argumentation. However, I want to be able to speak to people from other disciplines, particularly those in the humanities who study the ethics of RGTs. Therefore, I want to clarify some points that I have found from past experience to be a wellspring of misunderstanding between social scientists and other scholars. The primary misunderstanding concerns generalization. Consider a public opinion poll that you would read in the newspaper that says, "People in the South attend church more regularly than do people in the North." However, your brother lives in the South, and he never goes to church, so how could this statement be true? What the statement should actually say is that "on average" this statement is true. Social science is based on claims like this, and my book is no exception. I will repeatedly say in this book that "evangelicals tended to talk like this," or that "people I spoke with who used this discourse tended to approve of RGTs." These are generalizations, and there will be of course people I spoke with who do not fit the generalization. I may even not write the "tend to" after awhile, assuming we all understand the nature of the claims I am making.

Another disconnect with scholars in the humanities lies in the simplified social science depictions of concepts that are the focus of hugely detailed debates in the humanities. For example, in chapter 6, I devote approximately one page to describing an Irenean perspective on suffering, without even mentioning Irenaeus. I know that many books have been written on Irenean perspectives, but I make the barest of sketches—accurately, I hope. The reason that I do not go into great detail is that social science measurement devices are not precise enough to measure most concepts in such extreme detail. Social science methods are like sledgehammers, but they are the only tools that exist. That is why I use them.

Finally, the names of the respondents are fictional and other details have been changed to protect confidentiality. I also did not conduct all the interviews by myself, but relied on a team of research assistants; therefore, I use the first-person singular to describe my analysis and the first-person plural to describe the interviewing experience.

The History of Abortion, Reproductive Genetic Technologies, and the Contemporary Public's Views

In this chapter I delve deeply into the history of reproductive genetic technologies (RGTs) and more briefly into the history of the abortion debate. While I am primarily interested in the newer technologies, it is important to see how these new technologies evolved. The focus of this book is on how the ordinary religious person in the United States talks about RGTs, but this information is not always available historically.[1] Therefore, for this historical analysis of the technologies I must fall back on the reaction by religious elites like theologians and denominational officials. We can expect that religious elites' views to be at least somewhat related to the views of the members of their traditions because both groups are enmeshed in the same religious discourses. At the end of this chapter, I use the survey to examine the conclusions that the current religious public reaches about RGTs.

In the Beginning

Examining RGTs from "the beginning" to the present reveals two clear trends. The first is increasing precision. If the goal is, for example, to avoid having children with cystic fibrosis, this can be done more accurately today than in the past. The second trend is that in the past people who were not going to be the parents tried to determine the genetic qualities of children.

Today, any determination of the genetic qualities of children is going to be due to the autonomous decision-making of the parents.

It is important to make the obvious point that the technologies for RGT have existed for millennia. They just were not very accurate and involved mate selection or infanticide. It seems likely that people with obvious physical or mental problems—whether genetic or not—were considered to be unworthy mates, and newborns with obvious health problems were killed. Marrying into "the right" family also would presumably give the individual a modicum of control over the genetic characteristics of his or her children.

People, of course, had only a vague sense why children had physical features similar to their parents. The ancient Greeks thought that babies were the result of the "coagulation" of sperm and menstrual fluid, and both transmitted characteristics because both contained the "seed" contributed by all parts of the body that blended to produce the baby.[2] Even Charles Darwin, conducting research in the mid-nineteenth century, thought that there were invisible particles called "gemmules," which were in all the cells of organisms. The gemmules could be changed by the environment in which one was living, and the sperm and the egg were composites of these particles. This simply reinforced the dominant view at the time, that the characteristics of the offspring are "blended together to appear as an unpredictable mixture" of the traits of the parents.[3]

This ignorance began to recede with the research of Augustinian monk Gregor Mendel on the offspring of pea plants. When crossing plants grown from green and yellow seeds, the resulting plants were not a mixed color like brown, but rather yellow. Through careful experimentation, he discovered the concepts of dominant and recessive traits, and also determined that the plant received one "elemente" (as he called it) from each parent. We now call "elementes" are chromosomes, and humans receive one set from each parent. Although he published this work in 1865, it was more than thirty years before his work was recognized and continued.[4] This would become the building blocks for future genetic knowledge and, by extension, RGTs.

Mainline Eugenics

Although people had only the vaguest sense of how inheritance worked, they began to try to implement these ideas in social life through "improved" mate selection. In 1883 the term "eugenics" was coined by Francis Galton, an English scientist and cousin of Charles Darwin, to describe the science of this better breeding. Galton's goal in eugenics was to create a science of improving the human species by giving "the more suitable races or strains of blood a better chance of prevailing speedily over the less suitable."[5] That is, the "better" people should mate and have more children than the "inferior" people. This was the selection of the fittest applied to humans and not to pea plants.

Eugenics was necessary because, in the view of Galton and his British colleagues, modern inventions had made life easy, removing the imperative of the survival of the fittest. "Such measures as the minimum wage, the eight-hour day, free medical advice, and reductions in infant morality encouraged an increase in unemployables, degenerates, and physical and mental weaklings," Galton claimed. The result was, according to one of his colleagues, that natural selection had been replaced by "reproductive selection," which gave advantage "to the most fertile, not the most fit."[6]

What was considered to be "a more suitable race" or "strain of blood" was entirely wrapped in class prejudice. The eugenicists not only assumed that behaviors were inherited but also that one had only to look at the leaders of society, the intellectuals, artists, musicians, scientists, and members of the upper classes to see the result of good breeding. Criminality, "feeblemindedness," alcoholism, sexual immorality, and similar behaviors were considered to be undesirable and inherited genetic traits and, not coincidentally, found among the poor. The desire of early eugenicists was to increase the birthrate among the genetic "desirables" and to decrease it among the "undesirables."

In England, good inherited qualities were assumed to correspond with class lines. In the United States, not surprisingly given the nature of American society, they corresponded with race, nationality, or ethnicity. For example, American eugenicist Charles Davenport wrote in 1911 that the genes of Poles made them "independent and self-reliant though clannish," that the Italians tended toward "crimes of personal violence," and that the "Hebrews" were predisposed to "thieving," though rarely to personal violence.[7]

The American eugenics movement was intertwined with early-twentieth-century debates about immigrants, who were seen as the source of many social problems. If the social problems were caused by the genes of the immigrants, it would be a simple matter of progressive reform to not allow people with these genes into the country. Davenport, for example, thought that the new immigrants from eastern and southern Europe would make the American population "darker in pigmentation, smaller in stature, more mercurial . . . more given to crimes of larceny, kidnapping, assault, murder, rape and sex-immortality."[8]

In 1924, President Coolidge, who had earlier stated that "America must be kept American" because "biological laws show . . . that Nordics deteriorate when mixed with other races," signed an immigration control act designed to limit the immigration of persons from eastern and southern Europe.[9] This was then a crude type of RGT—controlling the genetic qualities of children by deciding who will be able to be in the same country, meet, marry, and bear children.

The Reform Eugenics Movement

Starting in the 1930s, there was increasing criticism that mainline eugenics was merely hidden class or race prejudice. Hermann Muller—one of the most influential eugenicists of the mid-twentieth century—wrote at the time that eugenics had become "hopelessly perverted" into a pseudo-scientific facade for "advocates of race and class prejudice, defenders of vested interests of church and state, fascists, Hitlerites, and reactionaries generally."[10]

The death knell to mainline eugenics was the revelation of the Nazi atrocities in Europe. Hitler was obviously the most famous follower of mainline eugenics with his notion of a "Nordic race" and "inferior races." In the words of historian Daniel Kevles, "a river of blood would eventually run from the [German] sterilization law of 1933 to Auschwitz and Buchenwald."[11] While one might think that revelation of Nazi atrocities would be the end of the very notion that some people are genetically not valuable to society, the Nazi revelations only delegitimated mainline eugenics, leaving reform eugenics in its place.

Reform eugenicists believed that there were valuable characteristics across all class and racial groups. They still wanted to "improve" the genetic quality of the entire population, but they had a more difficult challenge that they viewed as more scientifically legitimate: to identify those with "good" genes in any racial or ethnic group and encourage them to reproduce, and to discourage those with "bad" genes in any group to not reproduce.

While there were efforts at encouraging the "best" to breed more and the "undesirables" to breed less, the primary strategy was to limit the reproduction of what were seen as the extremely undesirable types through forced sterilization of the "feebleminded." State laws allowing this sterilization were passed in the early twentieth century, with one eventually resulting in the infamous 1927 *Buck v. Bell* Supreme Court case. In this case, which involved the sterilization of a seventeen-year-old "moral imbecile" named Carrie Buck, Justice Oliver Wendell Holmes concluded that sterilization was justified because "three generations of imbeciles are enough."[12]

The early-twentieth-century American eugenics movement was seen as a progressive social reform, as a way to "scientifically" solve social problems. This made it attractive to a contemporaneous religious movement—the Social Gospel, whose social location was primarily in what we would now call mainline Protestantism. The general idea was that Christians could bring on the second coming of Christ by creating the Kingdom of God on earth, and creating the Kingdom meant solving the social problems created by various aspects of modern industrial life. Many mainline Protestant clergy thus tried to convince their parishioners and the public to develop eugenic consciousness and then to not reproduce if they lacked "genetic fitness." Some clergy participated in eugenic sermon contests, and some tried to set up marriage certificate programs to certify the genetic health of those they married.[13] Liberal Jews, also active in social reform, participated with their Christian colleagues. While Catholics had their own version of social reform akin to the Social Gospel movement, they were generally opposed to eugenics because its methods, such as sterilization, violated church teachings.[14] Finally, evangelicals were not so much opposed to eugenics itself as they were to the underlying notion that clergy should be involved with social reform—in the evangelical world at that time, saving souls was the primary mission.

Religious advocacy on behalf of reform eugenics was then the result of a confluence of events, including the Social Gospel movement, theological modernism, and the popularity of "scientific" solutions.[15] It also seems likely that mainline Protestantism and Reform Judaism were supportive because they were white and middle- or upper-middle class, and the "fit" were always found in this group.

It was probably clear to all participants in the debate at the time that the use of state power for eugenic ends—even reform eugenic ends—was unlikely after the Holocaust. Even semicoercive measures, like the eugenic health certificates that would be required before being married in some mainline Protestant churches, were no longer viable, and the reform eugenicists now had to rely on free will. As Hermann Muller would say, people would have to realize that they had a "duty . . . to exercise their reproductive functions with due regard to the benefit or injury thereby done to society."[16] While some reform eugenicists like Muller were coming up with schemes to "improve" the gene pool by having "brilliant" men bank their sperm so it could later be implanted in women to increase the intelligence of the population, this never caught on.[17] What became more influential were efforts to avoid "damaging" the gene pool by engaging in "genetic counseling," that is, to convince those with genetic diseases to not have children themselves but to adopt. Controlling the genes of your offspring had become entirely voluntary, but precision remained extremely low.

Genetic Counseling

During this era, geneticists had made great strides in understanding the probabilities that children would inherit single-gene recessive diseases. Even in the 1950s, they could, through a family history, give a couple the probability that their children would have one of a limited number of diseases, such as sickle cell anemia, achondroplasia (a type of dwarfism), and cleft palate. This would eventually be called genetic counseling and was clearly intended originally to persuade certain people to not reproduce "for the good of the species." However, by the 1960s, people were criticizing this hold over of the eugenic "save the species" motivation, and soon it was accepted that counseling should focus on maximizing the happiness of the individual family and their offspring. For example, theologian John Fletcher would write in 1972—and clearly referencing the earlier links between the Social Gospel movement and reform eugenic thought—that people involved in this process of genetic counseling should "adhere to their therapeutic calling and resist any attempt to hasten the 'kingdom of God' through technical progress."[18] Rather, it should be the needs of the family, as understood by those family members, which should be the basis of reproductive decisions. Soon the dominant logic of genetic counseling was to provide good information to the potential parents, so that they could make their own autonomous decision as to whether to reproduce.

There was no obvious reaction within religious communities to the development of genetic counseling. To this day, the vast majority of religious communities do not oppose counseling whereby people decide whether to try to have a child, although some oppose the means by which you avoid having a child.[19]

Human Genetic Engineering

Returning to the postwar demise of mainline eugenics, tremendous strides in understanding the biochemical basis of genetic inheritance were occurring. Most notably, in 1953 Francis Crick and James Watson determined the chemical structure of DNA. Up until that point, scientists could simply look at features of the parents, look at the features of their offspring, and make an assessment that the offspring had or had not inherited a gene. How inheritance actually biochemically occurred was a mystery. After 1953, they could at least imagine that they could control the genes of the species by manipulating the genome.

It would take many years after 1953 for the details to be worked out. Yet, the fact that genetic inheritance had been reduced to biochemical reactions suggested to many the potential for a degree of precision in genetic control that was not possible with simply stopping people from having sex. Instead of encouraging people with desirable traits to have more children, many scientists were now dreaming of the day when genes with known functions could be "spliced" or "surgically repaired." If one could, for example, find *the* gene for intelligence, you could splice it into everyone's genome and eventually make the species more intelligent.

The ideas of the reform eugenicists were still driving this speculation. For example, one of the early conference proceedings debating human genetic engineering was titled "The Control of Human Heredity and Evolution,"[20] and the keynote address by Hermann Muller was titled "The Means and Aims of Human Genetic Betterment."[21] While some wanted to stop disease, others remained true to their eugenic forebears in advocating what we would now call enhancements. In 1963, Julian Huxley wrote that he wanted to use human genetic engineering to increase "man's desirable genetic capacities for intelligence and imagination, empathy and co-operation, and a sense of discipline and duty."[22]

For various reasons scientists pulled back from the reform eugenic vision in the 1970s to focus on what came to be known as somatic human genetic engineering, called somatic gene therapy by its proponents.[23] The technology is *not* reproductive. The genes of currently existing people would be repaired to resolve their diseases without affecting the genes of their reproductive cells.[24] More important, scientists never lost sight of the goal of influencing reproduction with human genetic engineering. This soon came to be called "germline" human genetic engineering, where the genes of a person's offspring (and all subsequent generations) would be changed.

To understand the current elite debates about RGTs, it is important to know that this original germline human genetic engineering debate from the 1950s to the early 1980s contained much religious discourse. The primary discourse was a variation on the "God and humanity" discourses (described in chap. 4), where the debate seemed to be over the proper role of humans in creation. Much of the elite theological opposition was focused on the idea that, because human genetic engineering influenced the genes of subsequent generations and thus the entire human species, this technology would be a case of humans "designing their own descendants." They also saw human genetic engineering, rightly, as a continuation of reform eugenic attempts by scientists to change the species.

In 1980, Jewish, Catholic, and mainline Protestant leaders wrote a letter to President Carter stating their concerns that human genetic engineering was "playing God," a letter which eventually resulted in a major report from a government bioethics commission.[25] Mainline Protestants also studied the issue extensively, with the National Council of Churches conducting multiple studies and statements, and some denominations, such as the United Methodist Church and the United Church of Christ, conducting their own studies. Outside these official channels, political activist Jeremy Rifkin organized groups of well-known denominational leaders and theologians to engage in various protests against human genetic engineering.[26]

Perhaps because this technology has not been achievable, theologians have actually not reached firm conclusions about its use. In general, they have supported somatic gene therapy, but reaction to germline human genetic engineering is more complicated. On the one hand, pretty much all religious elites have been opposed to enhancement human genetic engineering.[27] On the other hand, opinion is more mixed on health applications of human genetic engineering. During the last period when debate about germline human genetic engineering flared up, a range of denominational officials from across the theological spectrum, signed a public statement opposing all instances of human genetic engineering.[28] That said, mainline and liberal Protestants, as well as Jews, have not been categorically opposed to human genetic engineering for health applications, although they do not think human genetic engineering can be ethically applied at present. Catholic elites also are not categorically opposed to human genetic engineering for health applications if very stringent conditions could be met, such as the technology producing no harm to embryos, and not creating or manipulating embryos outside of the body.[29]

Conservative Protestants have been less clear about human genetic engineering for health applications, with only scattered statements from denominations and individual elites, but they have generally been negative. For example, in a recent collection of essays on the morality of human genetic engineering in different religious traditions, the one chapter written by conservative Protestants opposed human genetic engineering for enhancement *and health* applications.[30] (One of the authors is actually a well-known evangelical anti-RGT activist.)

Amniocentesis, Prenatal Genetic Testing, and the Abortion Debate

Returning again to the late 1960s, there was another development in reproductive genetic technology that would influence future debates. As of the mid-1960s, genetic counselors could only give couples probability statements about their children's possible genetic traits. For example, it was known that older women had a higher incidence of having children with Down syndrome. A decisive move toward increased precision occurred in 1967 with the development of amniocentesis. In this technology, a needle is inserted into the womb of a pregnant woman and some fluid is removed. This fluid, which contains cells from the fetus, is tested to determine the fetus's genetic characteristics, and fetuses with undesirable genetic qualities could be aborted.

For the first time, there was an exact test of the genetic qualities of offspring, although limited to very few conditions. Instead of a logic where certain types of people are stopped from encountering each other through immigration restrictions or by limiting marriage (mainline eugenics), instead of being sterilized or encouraged to not reproduce (reform eugenics), and instead of having their genetic problems "repaired" (the as of yet unobtainable human genetic engineering), amniocentesis introduced a new method where embryos and/or fetuses are created and then some of them are terminated on the basis of their genetic characteristics. This method would be influential in these debates from this point forward.

In the mid-1960s, abortion was illegal in all the states, with exceptions in some states for particular pregnancies, such as those that were the result of rape or incest. Nowhere was it solely a woman's choice.[31] In 1959, the American Law Institute had proposed a model penal code for states urging that abortion be legalized in the case of "substantial risk that continuance of the pregnancy would gravely impair the physical or mental health of the mother," if the fetus had a "grave physical or mental defect," or when the pregnancy is the result of rape or incest.[32] Some states began to enact these changes, with each abortion typically requiring the permission of a panel of doctors to ensure it fit the criteria.

Initially this liberalization of abortion law was not extremely controversial because these abortions were by definition rare, and the conditions that were being selected against were universally considered to be objectionable, such as Down syndrome. Put colloquially, amniocentesis followed by abortion was only available for "good" reasons. For example, in the early 1960s, the drug thalidomide caused severe deformations in babies when the pregnant woman took it during pregnancy. The case of a television personality in Arizona named Sherri Finkbine received public notoriety when, discovering that she had ingested thalidomide, and after being told by her doctor that she had a very high chance of having a child with severe birth defects, she attempted to get an abortion. She eventually went to Sweden to obtain an abortion, providing additional impetus to allow abortions in the United States for "good reasons" like undesirable conditions of the fetus.[33]

During this era, the leaders of the institutional Catholic Church were opposed to laws that made abortion more available, and organized efforts at opposing abortion liberalization were primarily organized by the Catholic Church. The official Catholic theology on this issue is fairly clear, at least in modern times—abortion was wrong from the moment of conception because it may be killing human life.

On the other hand, the leaders within mainline Protestantism became proponents of the liberalization of abortion laws. The motivations were to reduce the suffering of women facing difficult pregnancies and to promote what was portrayed as good scientific medical care, as well as to relieve the suffering caused by illegal abortion.[34]

An example of the advocacy by mainline Protestantism for the increased availability of abortion, particularly for "fetal defects," is the stance of the United Methodist Church. In 1968 this denomination was the second largest Protestant denomination in America, and it issued a "statement on responsible parenthood," which said that "we favor legislation on abortion along the lines recommended by the American Law Institute and the American Medical Association, allowing termination of pregnancy upon the recommendation of a qualified panel of physicians when it has been clearly determined that the physical or mental health of the mother is seriously threatened, or where substantial medical evidence indicates that a child will be born grossly deformed in mind or body, or where pregnancy has resulted from rape or incest."[35] Even the largest Protestant denomination, the more conservative Southern Baptist Convention, would, in 1971, "call upon Southern Baptists to work for legislation that will allow the possibility of abortion under such conditions as rape, incest, clear evidence of severe fetal deformity, and carefully ascertained evidence of the likelihood of damage to the emotional, mental, and physical health of the mother."[36] Although the Southern Baptists were officially in favor of the liberalization of abortion laws, by and large evangelicals and fundamentalists were not involved with this debate, making it a religious debate between mainline Protestants (and to a lesser extent Jews) and Catholics.

After attempts to reform abortion laws, attempts to make abortion even more widely available followed soon after, and mainline Protestants and Jews also were active in these efforts. The discourse used by the religious groups to argue for the further loosening of abortion laws was humanitarian—thousands of women were dying from illegal and unsafe abortions. This human need motivated a group of mainline Protestant and Jewish clergy during this era to start the Clergy Consultation Service on Abortion, which smuggled women for illegal yet safe abortions with reputable doctors and, in later years, to the states that had repealed their abortion laws.[37] Headed by an American Baptist pastor, the clergy network eventually spanned the country, although obviously without full coverage.

But of course religious groups were not the only groups interested in increasing access to abortion. Women's groups began to advocate for the repeal of all abortion laws, so that women could make their own decision without having to seek the approval from a panel of (typically male) doctors. This debate was sharply restructured by the 1973 *Roe v. Wade* Supreme Court decision, where the court ruled that state abortion laws were an unconstitutional infringement on the privacy of citizens. This created a new legal framework where states could regulate abortion for quality and safety before the end of the second trimester, but not try to limit it. In the third trimester of pregnancy, states could make abortion illegal, except when the health of the woman was at risk. The key was that it enshrined a particular argument about abortion into law: a balance between the state's interest in protecting fetal life and the privacy of women.

As is well known, the *Roe v. Wade* decision caught opponents of abortion off guard.[38] They could just not imagine that the debate would move from legalization in a few states to full-scale national legalization in one day. Immediately, opponents of abortion, led by the Catholic Church and organizations it had founded, began working for a constitutional amendment to overturn the *Roe v. Wade* decision, whereas liberal religious groups became defenders of abortion rights. For example, by 1976 the United Methodist Church statement on responsible parenthood had been modified and now included the clause that "we support the legal right to abortion as established by the 1973 Supreme Court decision.[39] Many of these liberal religious groups founded the Religious Coalition for Abortion Rights, a coalition of mainline Protestant denominations, Jewish movements, and other religious groups who all favored the *Roe v. Wade* decision.[40] The Religious Coalition for Abortion Rights included agencies of the American Baptist Churches, the Episcopal Church, the United Church of Christ, the United Methodist Church, the Christian Church (Disciples of Christ), and the predecessors to the Presbyterian Church (USA), as well as three of the four major Jewish movements and other religious groups.

A few years after the *Roe v. Wade* decision, we have the institutions in place for the abortion debate as it exists today. The liberal religious groups are still involved in the pro-choice side, but their advocacy is very small compared to the feminist women's organizations, Planned Parenthood, and the single-issue abortion rights organizations. On the pro-life side, the Catholic Church and the organizations it created were originally essentially the only organized opponents of abortion. Again, the central discourse of the Catholic Church concerning abortion has been consistent for over one hundred years; an embryo or fetus is human life, and to destroy it is wrong.

It is important to note that in the 1970s, evangelicals and fundamentalists were fairly uninvolved with politics and generally uninvolved with the abortion debate. Had they been active, it is fairly clear that they would have tended toward the conservative side of the debate (although the Washington representative of the Southern Baptist Convention helped found the Religious Coalition for Abortion Rights in 1973).[41]

However, looking at the official denominational statements about abortion among conservative Protestants over time, we see that if the abortion issue was raised before *Roe v. Wade*, or in the years immediately following *Roe v. Wade*, the reason for opposition to abortion was very often that abortion allowed for the concealment of sexual immorality by unmarried persons.[42] Public opinion research reports that this divide in reasoning between Catholics and conservative Protestants was represented in the views of ordinary religious persons. As two scholars of opinion over abortion write, "In the period immediately following the *Roe v. Wade* decision, Roman Catholics were more likely to oppose abortion out of respect for human life than because of traditional attitudes toward sexual morality, while the reverse pattern was observed among evangelical Protestants."[43]

This all changed in 1979 with the formation of the New Religious Right.[44] Evangelicals and fundamentalists lost their previous reticence to being active in politics and became involved in social movements concerning social issues like abortion, school prayer, the equal rights amendment, and so on. And, to put it simply, conservative Protestants adopted the Catholic arguments about life beginning at conception and slowly dropped arguments about sexual immorality. This too eventually was reflected in the views of ordinary religious persons. In public opinion, a number of years after the *Roe v. Wade* decision, the difference between Catholics and evangelicals, where Catholics are concerned about life and evangelicals about sexual morality, disappeared.[45] Since the early 1970s, in only twenty-five years, conservative Protestants have transformed themselves from a group that was somewhat opposed to abortion to the religious group that is the most opposed to abortion.[46] Within the religious community, the earlier conflict of mainline Protestants and Jews versus Catholics had, by the mid-1980s, changed to mainline Protestants and Jews versus Roman Catholics, evangelicals, and fundamentalists.

In Vitro Fertilization

Going back a bit in our historical narrative, the late 1960s were a time of great turmoil in human reproduction, although the connections were not obvious at the time. Abortion laws were being liberalized. Amniocentesis was invented. Scientists were claiming that human genetic engineering was near. And, in 1969 scientists in England created the first embryo in a test tube, the first step toward what is more technically known as a pregnancy through in vitro fertilization. The first baby born via in vitro fertilization did not occur until 1978.

In in vitro fertilization, a doctor removes eggs from a woman's ovaries and obtains sperm from a man. These two are placed together and the egg is fertilized. After it divides a few times and becomes a stable embryo, it is transferred to a woman's uterus. If implantation occurs, the woman carries the embryo to term for a normal pregnancy. This is a reproductive technology and not a reproductive *genetic* technology, because there was no way to influence the genes of the offspring, but its potential as a precursor to RGTs was identified even at the time of its invention.

The inventor of in vitro fertilization, embryologist Robert Edwards, writing one year after the successful creation of an embryo, mentioned that in vitro fertilization would help infertile parents have children of their own and went on to say that this research could lead to combining the genes either from two different animals or from different persons, which could lead to more precise genetic control.[47] In other words, he was fully embedded in the reform eugenic discourse of his era, and other reform eugenicists had anticipated these developments, with one arguing that in vitro fertilization could provide "a continuous, inexhaustible supply of the germ cells derived from selected male and female donors, carefully chosen on the basis of the demonstrated high quality of the children produced during their own lifetimes."[48]

These particular dreams of the eugenicists were put on indefinite hold because for many years the technology was only capable of facilitating regular reproduction. It could be used to bypass a blocked fallopian tube, but it could not help determine the genetic qualities of their offspring any more than by simply selecting with whom to mate (albeit a highly technological mating). This would eventually change.

The reaction of religious elites to in vitro fertilization is not as clear-cut as it was for abortion. The Roman Catholic Church is opposed to in vitro fertilization on multiple grounds. First, this technology often results in embryonic death, which is then unacceptable for the same reason that abortion is unacceptable. However, according to the Vatican, "even in a situation in which every precaution were taken to avoid the death of human embryos, homologous IVF . . . dissociates from the conjugal act the actions which are directed to human fertilization. For this reason the very nature of homologous IVF . . . also must be taken into account, even abstracting from the link with procured abortion."[49] That is, in vitro fertilization is wrong for the same reason contraception is wrong; it separates the unitative and procreative meaning of sexual activity.

On the liberal end of the spectrum, I am unaware of Jewish opposition to in vitro fertilization. In Judaism, embryos outside a woman's body do not have moral status, so embryonic destruction is not a moral problem. Mainline Protestant leaders have not been concerned with in vitro fertilization either, given that they have not been opposed to abortion. The more ambiguous group is evangelical Protestants, who, in regards to vitro fertilization, slightly part company with their Catholic allies in the antiabortion movement. Evangelicals are generally not opposed to contraception, as are Catholic elites, and lack the Catholic concept of the unitive purpose of sexual relations. One summary concludes that evangelicals "see IVF as a good solution for infertile couples who want children." However, "that acceptance is now coming under greater scrutiny because IVF clinics frequently discard 'excess' embryos."[50] As R. Albert Mohler, Jr., President of the Southern Baptist Theological Seminary, recently stated, "far too many evangelicals seem to turn a blind eye to this reality . . . While we celebrate the birth of a child and the gift of life, we cannot blind ourselves to the harsh and grotesque reality that this technology also means the destruction of human life."[51] In other words, evangelicals are not opposed to in vitro fertilization per se, but only to contemporary American practices that result in excess embryos. If the United States developed policies like those in Germany, where all created embryos must be implanted in the woman, in vitro fertilization presumably would not be opposed by evangelicals.[52]

Preimplantation Genetic Diagnosis: In Vitro Fertilization with the Logic of Amniocentesis

Using in vitro fertilization for reproductive genetic purposes had up to this point remained impossible. In 1990 a new RGT was invented that fused the technology of in vitro fertilization with the underlying logic of amniocentesis.[53] In preimplantation genetic diagnosis, a couple produces a number of embryos through in vitro fertilization, and each embryo is allowed to divide until it contains eight cells. At that point, one cell is removed and tested to determine its genetic qualities. Embryos with a genetic trait that the couple would like to avoid are discarded. Those that lack the trait to be avoided are implanted in the woman (so far it appears that removing this one cell does not negatively affect the children that are eventually born). This has the same logic of amniocentesis followed by abortion, but avoids the strain of the woman having to be pregnant and then having to potentially have an abortion. On the other hand, it requires in vitro fertilization, which is an expensive and potentially risky procedure, with a somewhat low rate of producing pregnancies.

Like amniocentesis, preimplantation genetic diagnosis started with screening embryos with genes for genetic diseases that would inflict great suffering on a child. However, when coupled with our increased ability to identify gene function, this technology can increasingly be used to screen for traits that are not universally considered to be diseases. For example, preimplantation genetic diagnosis can be used to avoid early-onset Alzheimer's disease or to select the sex of a child.[54] Although preimplantation genetic diagnosis has been discussed by religious leaders, it has been discussed primarily as part of the abortion debate, because of the inevitable embryonic destruction associated with the technique.

Another less invasive screening technique has been developed for one genetic trait—sex. It turns out that it is possible to separate X and Y chromosome sperm in a laboratory and only inseminate the woman with the desired type of sperm, coming close to guaranteeing that they will have a child of the desired sex. This is new enough that it has not been the subject of much discussion in the religious world.

Human Cloning

The most controversial RGT in recent years has been human cloning. There was a brief debate about this in the 1960s following the revelation that scientists in the 1950s and 1960s had succeeded in cloning frogs.[55] Another burst of debate came in the late 1970s after a book claimed to describe the cloning of a human, which was never demonstrated and later assumed to be a hoax.[56] This debate died down, probably because no mammals were cloned.

In 1997, scientists in Scotland announced the birth of "Dolly" the sheep, the first mammalian clone. To oversimplify, the DNA from an adult sheep cell was placed into an oocyte and tricked into thinking it was an embryo. It then began to divide and grow, like a normal embryo. People quickly assumed that it would soon be possible to clone a human. President Clinton announced a moratorium on government funding for cloning, and debate about cloning has continued to this day. One by one, additional mammals have been cloned, and in November 2007 cloning reached our close evolutionary relatives when it was announced that a cloned monkey embryo had been created.[57]

It is important to note some similar cloning terminology from yet another debate. I will only touch on this debate and not discuss it further in this book. Scientists have found that stem cells from embryos could potentially cure various diseases by being grown into useful tissues. To avoid the problem of rejection of unrelated tissues that would be implanted, some scientists have concluded that it would be most effective to create a cloned embryo from the person with the disease, but only allow the embryo to grow for a few days. The embryonic stem cells would be removed and used to heal the person with the disease. Some advocates of this technology have called this "therapeutic cloning." This is not reproduction and I will avoid talking about it further.

What we are talking about is "reproductive cloning," where the cloned embryo is transferred to the woman with the intention of producing a baby. Nothing in reproductive genetic technology has outraged the public like cloning, and all organized religious bodies that have taken official positions on reproductive cloning have opposed it.[58] In my analysis, with the exception of the religious traditions that are opposed to creating embryos outside of the womb in the first place (e.g., Catholicism), the reasons for opposition to cloning among religious leaders remain unclear.

Current Opinion

We can use the survey to get a sense of the likely conclusions about RGTs that will be reached by members of different religious groups. The first column in table 2 shows the degree of disapproval of various technologies for a random sample of all Americans.[59] Some basic patterns in the data are evident. First, if you look at the applications within each technology, as the application moves from avoiding fatal childhood diseases to increasing intelligence, there is increasing opposition along a disease-enhancement continuum. If you look at the same application accomplished via different technologies , you see that preimplantation genetic diagnosis is more opposed than prenatal testing and human genetic engineering is more opposed than preimplantation genetic diagnosis, although the effect of the technology is not as strong a determinant of approval as is the purpose of the application. There is also near-universal opposition to reproductive cloning.

The remaining columns show these same views for the high attenders of various religious traditions. In the survey, respondents could self-identify as follows: fundamentalist, evangelical, mainline, or liberal Protestant; or traditionalist, moderate, or liberal Catholic. The second to last

TABLE 2. **Respondents from Various Religious Traditions Disapproving of Reproductive Genetic Technologies (RGTs)**

| RGTs | Total all respondents | High attenders | | | | | | | Other religion |
| | | Protestants | | | | Catholics | | | |
		Fundamentalist	Evangelical	Mainline	Liberal	Traditionalist	Moderate	Liberal	
Prenatal testing									
To avoid a fatal childhood disease	27	42	46	21	20	46	30	17	36
To avoid adult onset disease	40	53	58	43	36	56	48	42	48
To determine sex	49	59	57	48	47	62	55	54	51
To select intelligence or strength in offspring	72	72	79	76	67	74	85	73	72
PGD									
To avoid a fatal childhood disease	32	52	57	32	23	52	37	36	43
To avoid adult onset disease	42	58	64	46	33	55	53	44	50
To determine sex	60	76	74	68	54	74	67	63	62
To select intelligence or strength in offspring	72	80	81	82	65	73	81	73	70
HGE									
To avoid a fatal childhood disease	43	59	67	42	37	57	41	47	49
To avoid adult onset disease	49	59	73	52	43	55	49	51	55
To determine sex	75	83	87	79	73	81	79	77	78
To select intelligence or strength in offspring	81	86	90	86	79	80	86	86	79
Reproductive Cloning	89	99	97	96	89	96	95	90	92

Note: Data are in percentages. PGD, preimplantation genetic diagnosis; HGE, human genetic engineering.

column is for respondents who regularly attend services that do not fit in the other categories. (This is a difficult to interpret mix of non-Christians and Christians who do not identify with the other traditions like Mormons and Eastern Orthodox.)

If we read across table 2, we see a pattern familiar to social scientists who study religion: fundamentalists, evangelicals, and traditional Catholics are the most opposed to these technologies, whereas mainline and liberal Protestants, as well as moderate and liberal Catholics, are less opposed. Of course, table 2 also disputes the idea that conservative religion in the United States is monolithic in its approach to social issues. For example, a majority of regular church-service–attending fundamentalists, evangelicals, and traditionalist Catholics are not opposed to abortion for a fatal childhood disease, and nearly half in each tradition are not opposed to using preimplantation genetic diagnosis for the same purpose. That said, religious conservatives are more opposed than others, and table 2 shows that opposition to RGTs is socially based in the conservative religious traditions in the United States. This demonstration of the conclusions that different people reach about these technologies is only the first step toward understanding opposition to RGTs and the effectiveness of a future debate. To more deeply understand, we must see how people justify their opposition, a task we turn to next.

CHAPTER THREE

Talking about Embryonic Life

In this chapter I introduce the embryonic life discourse, which is the primary discourse used to oppose abortion in the United States. The embryonic life discourse is important because so many people use it to oppose a range of reproductive genetic technologies (RGTs). However, I will not dwell on showing how the embryonic life discourse is used because it will be discussed in length in the next three chapters and because it is one of the best known discourses in the public sphere.

This section of the book focuses on not only showing the discourses that are used to oppose RGTs but also on evaluating the possibility of deliberation about RGTs across the abortion divide. In this chapter I will concentrate on evaluating whether people who oppose abortion for cystic fibrosis using the embryonic life discourse—the pro-lifers—*only* use that discourse. If so, then RGTs that do not destroy embryos would not be talked about like abortion, and the concerns about a merged abortion and RGT issue are misplaced. RGTs would not be perceived to be part of the abortion issue, and there would be no concerns about a lack of debate about RGTs.

Lack of Argumentative Complexity and the Abortion Issue

Existing scholarship suggests that pro-lifers may only use the embryonic life discourse to oppose abortion. With the language of absolutes that has developed in the debate, you only logically need one discourse because each side makes a fundamental claim. To quote from the bumper-sticker versions of the two sides, to be "pro-life" means that you believe that an embryo or a fetus is a "life" of equivalent moral standing as a born person; therefore, to destroy such life is wrong, even murder. To be "pro-choice" means that you believe that it is a part of women's fundamental rights to decide about the morality of abortion for themselves; therefore, abortion has to be broadly available. It is well established that these are the two dominant discourses in the abortion debate.[1]

It has been found that compared to discourse about other issues in the public sphere, the discourse of antiabortion and pro-choice organizations scores low in "integrative complexity," meaning that rigid black-and-white argumentation is dominant.[2] Sociologist Michele Dillon speculates that this is due to the abortion debate being a "clash of worldviews"; thus, the low complexity may be attempts by activists to not acknowledge the legitimacy of the views of people with the alternative worldview.[3] Moreover, the positions of some of the actors do not lend themselves to multiple arguments. For example, Dillon concludes that the position of the Catholic Church's "antiabortion position is absolute and inflexible . . . Since opposition to abortion constitutes a core, non-negotiable tenet of Catholic teaching, reflecting its privileging of a monolithic right to life, it is reasonable, in the absence of previous research, to expect the Church to argue its case in an integratively simple way. From an impression management perspective, integratively simple statements that present issues in unambiguous black-and-white terms communicate commitment and firmness of resolve, whereas integratively complex statements communicate an openness to compromise"[4]

Other scholars also have concluded that this lack of integrative complexity that results in black-and-white discourse (like the sole use of the embryonic life discourse) has trickled down to ordinary citizens. A study of public opinion over time concludes that what the authors consider to be the arguments of the antiabortion movement, attitudes toward sexuality and belief about the sanctity of life, are being used more now than in the past.[5]

Some intellectuals who are in favor of expanding the opposition to abortion domain to include RGTs also see ordinary persons as only using the embryonic life discourse; therefore, they think that ordinary people will be unable to see all RGTs as part of a broader issue that includes abortion. For example, Leon Kass is a secularly oriented conservative thinker who is well regarded by religious conservatives. He was a Professor of Social

Thought at the University of Chicago, the Chair of the President's Council on Bioethics during the presidency of George W. Bush, and a Fellow at the American Enterprise Institute. He has made an impassioned plea for evangelicals and other religious conservatives to move beyond their concerns with embryonic life. He does not want them to abandon these concerns, but rather to address "additional threats to human dignity," by which he meant RGTs. After recalling the introductory pages of the novel *A Brave New World* where the reader is given a tour of the incubation room where the clones are passing by in bottles, Kass said that it would be a shame if religious conservatives shrugged their shoulders at the decanting of the first clone because no embryos were hurt in the process.[6] Kass would later write that "certain pro-lifers appear to care little whether babies are cloned or even 'born' in bottles, so long as no embryo dies in the process."[7] Kass wants "pro-lifers" to expand to opposing RGTs like cloning, but is worried that they only use the embryonic life discourse and thus lack another discourse that could be used to oppose cloning.

Similarly, Nigel M. de S. Cameron is an evangelical intellectual who has been involved with trying to form coalitions between liberal and conservative critics of RGTs. He was Provost and Distinguished Professor of Theology and Culture at Trinity Evangelical Divinity School, and is currently the President of the Institute on Biotechnology and the Human Future at Chicago-Kent College of Law. He shares a similar concern with Kass and also uses cloning as the exemplar case, writing that pro-lifers "have been less certain of what would actually be wrong if the technique [of reproductive cloning] were perfected . . . and it became as 'safe' as in vitro fertilization, or maybe even as safe as natural pregnancy." He specifies additional discourses to use in opposing abortion: the Promethean fatalist discourse (see chap. 4) and the individual dignity/equality discourse (described in chap. 5). He calls this a broader agenda for the "more complex threat to the dignity of humankind [that] lies on the horizon":

> Abortion is not, ultimately, about just the killing of the unborn; it is about the power to kill—the power of some human beings over others, the power of the born over the unborn, the unbridled power of one generation to make life and death decisions about the next. Abortion kills the unborn, but not as an end in itself. It kills them in order to demonstrate that mothers and fathers and doctors and the courts will always have the final say in determining the life of the unborn. It kills them to underline our ultimate authority over the generation to come.

He then wants to apply the discourses that he advocates for use with opposition to abortion to opposition to RGTs. The intent of the new technologies is, he continues, "to give us control—not through the primitive barbarism of aborting the unborn, but through the new, sophisticated barbarism of designing the born. . . . this new kind of crime does not simply destroy people made in God's image; it makes people in our own."[8] Cameron wants to shift the conversation about stopping abortion away from solely using the embryonic life discourse to simultaneously using other discourses that can be used to argue against both abortion and the new technologies. He, too, is obviously concerned that "pro-lifers" only use the embryonic life discourse. Of course, whether opponents of abortion only use the embryonic life discourse to oppose abortion for cystic fibrosis is an empirical question.

Opposing Abortion for Cystic Fibrosis

The in-depth interviews conducted for this book had an intentional progression of topics (for a copy of the interview guide, see the Religious Respondent Interview Guide). After a number of preliminaries, the interviewer and interviewee discussed whether a hypothetical couple should have an abortion after amniocentesis determined that the fetus the woman was carrying had cystic fibrosis. We then discussed preimplantation genetic diagnosis for cystic fibrosis, which was followed by preimplantation genetic diagnosis for a series of conditions each more distant from health concerns and more toward enhancement. After a discussion of sperm sorting for sex, the series of conditions started again, but with the technology being human genetic engineering. These questions ended with a discussion of cloning. I use this order of questions in the interview to structure the claims I make.[9]

Consistent with the history of abortion discourse, the survey used in this book (table 2), and countless surveys by social scientists, interviewees from liberal religious groups tend to argue that abortion for cystic fibrosis is an acceptable alternative, and members of conservative traditions are less likely to make this case. Few Jews thought abortion for cystic fibrosis was wrong, and liberal and mainline Protestants, as well as people who identified themselves as liberal Catholics, were slightly more conservative than Jews. Evangelicals, fundamentalists, and self-identified traditionalist Catholics were the most likely to say that abortion was always or almost always wrong, including in the case where the fetus has cystic fibrosis. Of course, there were strongly pro-choice evangelicals and strongly pro-life liberal Protestants—these traditions are not monolithic.

The most consistently used discourse to oppose abortion for cystic fibrosis *was* the embryonic life discourse. For example, when we asked Phil, a traditional evangelical, about amniocentesis for cystic fibrosis, he said that this is obviously a "difficult question, the foundations of what it means to value life, are in part innately human and part for those who are Christians, they have spiritual values as well. So, from a human standpoint, I can see how that would be a very difficult position to be in, and any family who is getting started, would have a struggle with that question." Despite seeing the situation as difficult, he clearly has a conclusion, which is that the couple should just continue the pregnancy because abortion is wrong.

He most clearly articulates his embryonic life discourse when discussing preimplantation genetic diagnosis. After clarifying what preimplantation genetic diagnosis entails, he uses the embryonic life discourse, saying: "I see what you mean. . . . That is a unique circumstance, but with my belief that life begins at conception, I would have great difficulty with that process and I would not pursue it. . . . life begins at conception and that you are breeding four lives to choose one and let the three others go away. I don't give myself that freedom to make those choices." When the interviewer asked whether preimplantation genetic diagnosis would be better than amniocentesis, he said:

> I don't see it as a difference, because again the way I see the definition from a moral standpoint that life begins at conception and that gives responsibilities to all parties ahead of that event to be prepared for the responsibility of that, so I can't endorse either option as I said before. Abortion would be a horrible option for the child as would this other method, even though you have eight cells.

Phil has clearly talked about the situation of abortion before, and uses the embryonic life discourse for that situation. When he encounters the new situation of preimplantation genetic diagnosis, that new situation seems analogous to abortion to him ("I don't see it as a difference"), so he also uses the embryonic life discourse for this new situation. For Phil, the opposition to abortion domain already includes preimplantation genetic diagnosis.

Margaret is similar to Phil. She would recommend amniocentesis to
test for cystic fibrosis, but only to obtain the genetic information and not
to use that information to have an abortion. She said:

> Well, then maybe I would want to know so that I could be prepared so that if it
> was; I would get my hands on all the research that I could; I would find the best
> facility and the best doctors I could so I could make sure that from the time that
> child was born, it would have every opportunity to have the best life possible;
> the healthiest life but I could not abort. I couldn't do that.

So, why not abort? she was asked. "Because it's a breathing, living being. It's a person," she replied. After using a number of the discourses,
which we will examine in later chapters, she returns to use the embryonic life discourse while discussing preimplantation genetic diagnosis by
saying:

> My understanding is they might implant four but then she can decide later on
> to abort three, if they only want one child, and it's a living being. And so that's
> a problem. . . . And that's what [the doctor is] doing basically, in the lab, he's
> deciding which ones to keep and which ones to throw out, it's a living and a life
> force.

She then uses a number of phrases popularized by the right-to-life movement, that "it's just an innocent life even though it can't breathe, even
though it doesn't have a beating heart, they've created a life." When asked
if preimplantation genetic diagnosis was better than amniocentesis, she returned to the embryonic life discourse after having used other discourses:

> No because for the reason . . . then you have these . . . they'd have to make a
> decision about these lives that they've chosen not to implant or once they have
> implanted and the woman decides she only wants a single pregnancy and you
> know there would still be other lives that they have created.

For Margaret, as with Phil, the opposition to abortion domain depicted
on the left side of figure 3 has already expanded to include preimplantation genetic diagnosis, even though this is the first time they had heard of
preimplantation genetic diagnosis.

I will not belabor the point that a certain portion of particularly the
conservative religious community uses this discourse to oppose abortion

for cystic fibrosis, because that is well known. What is more interesting is whether the exclusive use of this discourse for abortion constrains how the other RGTs are discussed.

Respondents Who Use Only the Embryonic Life Discourse

The discussions with the pro-lifers who only use the embryonic life discourse show how this exclusive use would preclude the merger of the abortion issue with RGTs that do not result in embryonic death. Unlike most other pro-lifers who use the embryonic life discourse to discuss abortion or preimplantation genetic diagnosis, these people *only* use the embryonic life discourse and, when embryonic life no longer fits by analogy to the new issue (because embryos are not involved), either say they were opposed and cannot say why, or state their opposition using a discourse that they do not and probably could not use to also talk about abortion (e.g., the RGT is not safe). More extreme were people who, once realizing that their embryonic life discourse did not fit, approved of any technology they encountered, because they lacked discourses to oppose the new situations. Any of these scenarios will limit merger because different discourses would be used for the new issues than would be used for abortion.

To see how the sole use of the embryonic life discourse would limit the merger of abortion and RGTs, let us look at our interview with Lisa, a middle-aged business woman who attends a nontraditional evangelical church. A former Sunday school teacher, she is quite active, attending services and Bible studies weekly. In the first scenario, we discussed a woman who is pregnant and a carrier for cystic fibrosis. Should she have amniocentesis to see if the fetus has the condition, and if so, have an abortion? Lisa was like a good portion of the evangelicals, saying "it wouldn't matter whether the baby has it or not. I'm 100% against abortion so I don't think that's a reason to take a life of a child." The equating of "fetus" with "child" suggests use of the embryonic life discourse. Unlike others we will meet in subsequent chapters, she does not use additional discourses at this point to say why abortion for cystic fibrosis would be wrong.

The next scenario was preimplantation genetic diagnosis for cystic fibrosis, and she said she would advise the hypothetical couple to not consider it, saying: "Once you fertilize an egg with the sperm, you have— we don't know exactly what you have. Until we can absolutely determine when life begins, I think it's way too cavalier of us to take that life. So once fertilization has happened, to me, it's not an option anymore. That's a life and it has every right to come to full term." While perhaps not as certain as evangelical leaders would like her to be about the status of an embryo, clearly she is on the right to life side, and generally using the embryonic life discourse.

Later we asked about the hypothetical couple named "Andy and Anne." They really want to have a girl and want to use preimplantation genetic diagnosis to find the female embryos to transfer to Anne's uterus and to dispose of the male embryos. Lisa continued in her clear use of the embryonic life discourse saying, "There will be no reason that I think they should make fertilized eggs and then throw away the ones they don't want to use because there's a chance that those are lives." Again, she seems to be upholding a slight derivation of the embryonic life discourse, that is, we are not sure if embryos are people, so we should "err on the side of life." Of course, the embryonic life discourse is logically sufficient to oppose these technologies, but, unlike others, she uses no other discourses. Preimplantation genetic diagnosis *is* part of the opposition to abortion domain for Lisa, because she uses the same embryonic life discourse to oppose both abortion and preimplantation genetic diagnosis.

For the next question, she was asked whether it was okay to use sperm sorting instead of preimplantation genetic diagnosis to obtain a female baby. Her response was that "I think that's okay. . . . I do. You're not taking a life that's already started. You're messing around with it, with the process a bit. But you're messing around with the process with birth control and all sorts of other things. That, to me, is not wrong." This is a separate issue for her, analogous to the issue of birth control that she has clearly discussed in the past. Abortion is only about embryonic life, and this new issue does not invoke embryonic life, so it is not the same as abortion. As I will note in subsequent chapters, many of her fellow evangelicals use other discourses to state their opposition to sperm sorting. But for Lisa, because no embryos were damaged in this case, it was fine.

When it came time to discuss human genetic engineering to remove or repair the gene for cystic fibrosis, which we portrayed as not harming embryos, Lisa had little to say, replying that:

I'm okay with that if there's no taking of any lives of embryos. Yes, it would just be altering and fixing that one that is fertilized. Yes, I think that's okay. . . . if there was a way they could get rid of cancer and Alzheimer's and Parkinson's. My [close relative][10] has Parkinson's. And all these diseases, gosh, I don't see a problem with that. And really what you're doing is treating a human being. They just happen to be in utero or in a test tube or whatever they're in. I certainly am not opposed to treating human beings for diseases.

She saw human genetic engineering for obesity no differently, because you would also treat a born person for obesity. She objected to human genetic engineering for intelligence because it removes variety in persons:

> Now you're really messing with the richness of life. Intelligence is not, even low intelligence, to me, is not a horrible thing. Granted, it can cause embarrassment or it can cause all sorts of things but there are a lot of low intelligent people that have wonderful lives and again, add to the richness of our experience.

On this application that does not harm embryos, she is opposed, but uses a discourse that is not used to oppose abortion; thus, there would be no shared discourse between abortion and human genetic engineering and therefore no new domain that includes abortion. Finally, almost nobody approves of cloning. Lisa is more ambiguous because of her sole dependence on the embryonic life discourse. She says cloning is:

> LISA: Way over the line, in my opinion. First of all, from what I'm hearing about cloning, yes, you inject the- what did you say? You inject [what]?"
>
> INTERVIEWER: A cell from somebody's skin is put into a woman's egg and then made to start growing.
>
> LISA: Okay, into a woman's egg that's already fertilized?
>
> INTERVIEWER: And then the embryo that grows from this event is then put into a woman's uterus.
>
> LISA: Okay, I've been told that when that is injected into the egg, the egg is already fertilized and you actually take the nucleus out of a fertilized egg and put this nucleus in. In that case, I'm opposed to it because you're already talking about a fertilized egg that's starting to grow. If you're not talking about that and I don't know enough about cloning to know, if you're just putting the skin cell into an egg that is not fertilized yet, I don't have nearly as much a problem with it for those reasons.

Lisa wants to know, to paraphrase Kass's evocative statement, whether any embryos will be hurt when the first clone is decanted. If not, then she "doesn't know enough about cloning to know." Lisa clearly only uses this one discourse and with only this discourse she is not opposed to RGTs that do not harm embryos. If Lisa were representative of most users of the embryonic life discourse, we could say that merger of the abortion and RGT issues would stop at preimplantation genetic diagnosis (because it kills embryos) and the creation of a new opposition to genetic control domain that includes the other RGTs and abortion is impossible.

Similarly, Betty is a middle-aged woman who works in child care and attends a traditional evangelical church. When we asked her about amniocentesis as an option, she used the embryonic life discourse, saying, "that is a child, to me, whether you test or not. You are pregnant and you need to have the baby. So, for me, in that scenario, the abortion option is not an option. There is nothing you can do, because that is murdering a life." When asked about preimplantation genetic diagnosis for cystic fibrosis, she continued in her exclusive use of the embryonic life discourse. She said this was wrong: "Simply because my personal view is that from the moment of conception that is a life. If it is eight cells or millions of cells, it is . . . granted it is not viable, it cannot live outside the womb kind of life, but to me that is where you draw the line with that. You have to draw the line."

She ruled out other uses of preimplantation genetic diagnosis on the same grounds. In other words, her opposition to abortion domain has expanded to include the new issue of preimplantation genetic diagnosis. When asked about sperm sorting, she simply said, "That would be fine." When asked if it was better than preimplantation genetic diagnosis, she said, "Oh, yes . . . simply because you are not . . . you are not dealing with a human life there. You know, until it is joined to the egg and starts making a life, it is just a sperm. I don't have a problem with that." When asked whether she has any other concerns with this sperm-sorting technology, she said the only concern she could think of was that "it takes all the fun out of it."

When our conversation turned to human genetic engineering for cystic fibrosis, she concluded that she "did not have a problem with that." Having used the embryonic life discourse that she shares with many of her fellow evangelicals, she does not use any of the other concerns voiced by evangelicals, but rather comes up with one of the discourses used by nearly everyone, saying she is concerned "about the risks . . . the risk to the mother, the risk to the child, any time there is a procedure, that would be my only concern." When we discussed human genetic engineering for obesity, she was supportive:

> Because obesity can create a whole bunch of medical problems later in life, even early in life. Obese children have a lot of medical problems, diabetes and

things like that and if changing that gene to prevent obesity, to me that is a health thing. If they wanted somebody with blue eyes instead of brown eyes, then I would say, "You are taking this a little bit too far," but I don't have a problem with that.

In the next question, we had an opportunity to discuss what she considered to be "too far" when we asked about human genetic engineering for intelligence. Her objection was that it was not worth the effort:

BETTY: I think that is silly. I really do. I mean, you know, I think that is just like . . . you are going too far. [*Laughter*] . . . I don't know, to me that is silly. I don't know why anybody would even think about doing that. To me it is so unnecessary.

INTERVIEWER: Some people might think that it would be good to give a child more intelligence, or as much intelligence as possible.

BETTY: I think intelligence is overrated. I think if you could give them common sense, to me that would be far more important than high intelligence. Because, intelligence is not a guarantee of a happy life or a success, or wisdom, you know, just because somebody is smart, to me, and somebody else is not as smart, that is silly. I think that is kind of putting too much of emphasis on that particular trait. There is a value to all different levels of intelligence.

While this is a discourse of opposition—albeit one not often used by respondents—it clearly is not one that would also be used to also oppose abortion. In sum, Betty also represents a singular focus on the embryonic life discourse that would hamper the merger of the issues of abortion, preimplantation genetic diagnosis, and the RGTs that do not harm embryos. In later chapters we will see whether the range of discourses that are used to oppose abortion are also used to oppose the range of new RGTs.

Prevalence of Using Only the Embryonic Life Discourse for RGTs

We can use the survey to get an estimate of the percentage of religiously active pro-lifers who do not use the other discourses found in subsequent chapters. The survey asked questions that measure the willingness of the respondent to use the embryonic life, Promethean fatalism, individual dignity/inequality, and meaningful suffering discourses to oppose RGTs in general.[11]

TABLE 3. **Use of Primary Oppositional Discourses by the Pro-life, Strongest Opponents of Reproductive Genetic Technologies Who Frequently Attend Religious Services**

Discourse	Percentage
Does not use Promethean fatalist discourse	8
Uses Promethean fatalist discourse	92
Does not use individual/dignity equality discourse	10
Uses individual dignity/equality discourse	90
Does not use meaningful suffering discourse	13
Uses meaningful suffering discourse	87
Does not use all three discourses	26
Uses all three discourses	74

The respondents whose responses are summarized in table 3 are the stronger opponents of RGTs who use the embryonic life discourse. They are also people who attend services regularly, making them roughly equivalent to the in-depth interviewees.[12] In this rendering of the data, only 8 percent of those who use the embryonic life discourse do not use the Promethean fatalist discourse to oppose RGTs in general, with slightly higher percentages for the other two discourses. While the in-depth interviews suggest that this sort of person, if prevalent, would stop the formation of a new domain that includes abortion and RGTs that do not harm embryos, the survey suggests that this sort of person is fairly rare.

Table 3 can also provide basic information about whether the pro-lifers also use the discourses I identify in the next three chapters to oppose RGTs. The table shows that 92 percent of pro-life opponents of RGTs also use the Promethean fatalism discourse to oppose some RGT, and similar percentages are found for the other two discourses. This means that the respondents use these three distinct discourses at some point, suggesting they have a broader repertoire of discourses with which to discuss both abortion and RGTs. In fact, a strong majority (74 percent) of pro-lifers also use all three of the other discourses. This suggests that these three discourses could comprise a unified discourse for a broader issue domain that encompasses both abortion for cystic fibrosis and RGTs. The use of these three discourses is associated with greater opposition to RGTs.[13]

While surveys can be used to evaluate the prevalence and representativeness of discourses in a population, they have limitations. This survey only shows that the respondent uses these discourses for RGTs in general.

It cannot show which RGT they are using them for, whether they also use them for abortion, or whether these discourses are salient enough that they would use them if they were not prompted by the survey. To look at these missing pieces of information, we will more closely examine the in-depth interviews beginning in the next chapter.

Nature, God, Humanity, and Promethean Fatalism

The fight against the naturalistic fallacy was supposed to be over. One of the great achievements of modern philosophy was to undermine arguments from Nature. No longer would educated people argue that homosexuality, powered flight, and the education of women were *unnatural*. . . . Montaigne's plea "Let us give Nature a chance; she knows her business better than we do"—was either to be decisively rejected or to be labeled "religious" (which amounted to the same thing in a rationalistic world). If this was the plan, it did not survive contact with the enemy.—James Boyle[1]

This chapter is ultimately about nature, and analysis of the interviews shows that most of the people with whom we spoke had a discourse about nature that they used to oppose some instances of reproductive genetic technologies (RGTs). However, for a subset of people, nature had a more theological meaning, specifically that God made nature or has intentions in nature. So, while most people speak of nature, these more theological discourses about God and nature are critical for understanding how the religious citizens talk about RGTs.

I have two goals in this chapter. First, I explore the variety of discourses used by both the strong opponents and (relative) proponents of RGTs that focus on the concepts of nature, God, and humanity. In addition to the general discourse about "nature," as well as the specific Promethean fatalist discourse I have mentioned in earlier chapters, I also describe the related discourses of natural law and hubris. I find that Promethean fatalism *is* used by the strongest opponents of RGTs, and the other discourses used by the (relative) proponents. My second goal is to examine whether the oppositional discourse of Promethean fatalism is used by the pro-lifers to oppose both abortion and RGTs, which would contribute to a merger of the issues. I also determine whether the pro-lifers and the non–pro-lifers use the Promethean fatalist discourse, which tells us whether a conversation about RGTs could cross the abortion divide. As in each of the next three chapters, I begin by examining academic discussions about these discourses to better understand them and what is at stake in their use by respondents.

The Naturalistic Fallacy

From our conversations with the interviewees it is clear that almost everyone assumes that what is "natural" is good. This is pervasive in our everyday lives, as one trip to the store will attest, with the claims of "natural" fibers and "natural" food. Gay Becker, in her study of people who use RGTs, similarly concluded that people have a strong preference for "the natural" way to reproduce and that they do not consider reproductive technologies to be "natural."[2] I found the same to be true with the people we interviewed.

But, should we allow what is "natural" to determine what is ethical? David Hume, philosopher of the eighteenth-century Scottish Enlightenment, was an opponent of deriving prescriptive statements (what ought to be) from descriptive statements (what is).[3] This has come to be known as the "is-ought problem" or the closely related "naturalistic fallacy" (the fallacy being that you can derive what to do from nature). In ethical claims about RGTs, the naturalistic fallacy occurs when someone claims that a way of making babies is or is not ethically acceptable purely because it is or is not "natural."

Bioethicists and philosophers are generally opposed to following nature.[4] Social scientists also have been early and frequent critics of the argument that some social practice cannot be changed because it is "part of nature" and is thus supposed to be that way. This is because, as social scientists point out, "nature" is not objective; rather, what we think is the "nature" that we should follow largely depends on one's social location. This is not a new critique. For example, in the nineteenth century, Friedrich Engels commented on the social Darwinism of his day, which was purported to be a law of nature, by saying,

the whole Darwinist teaching of the struggle for existence is simply a transfer-
ence, from society to living nature, of Hobbes's doctrine *bellum omnium con-
tra omnes*[5] and of the bourgeois-economic doctrine of competition, together
with Malthus's theory of population. When this sleight of hand has been per-
formed . . . the same theories are transferred back again from organic nature
into history, and it is now claimed that their validity as eternal laws of human
society has been proved.[6]

With this insight in mind, the social science list of once "natural facts"
now considered to be ideologies is quite long. Most relevant for this book
is the eugenics movement, which claimed that nature's laws revealed
that people of certain ethnicities were genetically predisposed to thiev-
ery, sloth, and so on—a view now recognized as race and class prejudice
transferred to nature. The social science consensus is that we should not
see nature as an external objective entity that can independently inform
our ethics, but rather we should understand the definition of nature as a
type of cultural formation.[7] Social scientists are then inclined to see claims
about nature as a strategy used to impose views, recognizing that the best
way for a person to institutionalize their claims is to establish that the
phenomenon in question is "natural."[8]

Following Natural Law

We then have hypothetical endpoints of a continuum between, on one end,
following nature and, on the other, considering nature to not be a meaningful source of ethics. The religious versions of the relationship with nature
fall in between and depend on a more complicated relationship among
God, humans, and nature. In contrast to the mainstream of philosophy,
bioethics, and social science, there are still many academics who disagree
that there is a naturalistic fallacy. The most influential contemporary theory of how to follow nature is natural law theory, a set of ideas that can be
found among the ancient Greeks, most notably Aristotle, as well as among
medieval Jewish, Islamic, and Christian theologians. In Catholic thinking,
natural law is associated with St. Thomas Aquinas and the Thomist school
of philosophy. While having an old and diverse pedigree, natural law theology became even more clearly associated with the Catholic tradition after
the release of the papal encyclical *Humanae vitae* in 1968, which famously
used natural law to argue that birth control was illicit.[9]

John Haldane argues that the common misunderstanding of natural law theory is that acting "in accord with nature" is "a recommendation of general noninterference, or of letting what will happen happen." This is fatalism and is located at one of the hypothetical endpoints I discussed above. However, Haldane argues that a true natural law theory is in the middle of the continuum, where the natural is "that which ought to be, not merely that which happens to be." For example, the Catholic natural law view of contraception is that "therapeutic medical interventions are warranted because they are aimed at protecting or restoring normal functioning; while contraceptive intervention is improper because it is intended to inhibit or destroy proper functioning."[10] How "proper functioning" is determined is an enormous debate in Catholic ethics, but for our purposes, it is enough to know that there is a school of thought that says that what we "ought" to do on issues of reproduction can be derived from the "is" of the *true nature* of the human.

Catholic theologians are not the only ones who believe that the "is" of what human beings are can determine the "ought" when it comes to RGTs. Bioethics has recently split into what Arthur Caplan calls the "left-liberal" wing and the "alliance of neo-conservative and religiously oriented bioethicists."[11] While the "left-liberals" could almost be defined by their opposition to the naturalistic fallacy, many of the neoconservative bioethicists are committed to deriving the "ought" from the "is" of nature.[12] Francis Fukuyama, a prominent figure who was a commissioner on the President's Council on Bioethics, writes that "the common understanding of the naturalistic fallacy is itself fallacious and that there is a desperate need for philosophy to return to the pre-Kantian tradition that grounds rights and morality in nature."[13] He approvingly cites attempts to define the natural human that could be used to determine the limits of RGTs, like one that lists "twenty natural desires that are universals characterizing human nature."[14] He ultimately defines the true human nature that should guide us as "the sum of the behavior and characteristics that are typical of the human species, arising from genetic rather than environmental factors."[15]

Hubris Versus Prometheus

There are additional religiously oriented discourses that have been identified or promoted by academics that fall between the hypothetical extremes and focus on the responsibilities of God and humans in nature. There is God, as well as nature, and the people who were created by God. Determining the responsibilities of God and humans has been a central theme in academic and theological discourse about RGTs.[16] There are many religious discourses that address this issue, with most of the Christian discourses having a high degree of overlap. For example, they would all agree on the idea that humans are not God.

In an extremely insightful article, Patrick Hopkins makes a distinction between the "hubris" objection to technology and the "Promethean" objection—essentially two different discourses about the relationship between God and humans concerning nature.[17] The hubris objection focuses on "the sheer audacity of human beings to go where only God has gone before." The basic idea here is that "human pride leads to moral and metaphysical overreaching—a sinful attempt to intrude on power and knowledge that belong to God alone, or a pathetic claim to be equal to God."[18] In the Christian tradition, there are two dominant stories that illustrate hubris: the Fall and the Tower of Babel. In the Fall, "to avoid the limitations set on her by God, Eve disobeyed God" and ate from the tree of knowledge so that she and Adam could become "like Gods." She and Adam were subsequently expelled by God from Eden.[19] In the Tower of Babel narrative, the people tried to build a tower that would reach the heavens to try "to be like God." God foiled their plans by making everyone speak a different language, causing construction to stop. To continue the metaphor to an RGT, the human attempt to clone is akin to our trying to be God. Hopkins writes that the traditional hubris criticism

> focuses on moral failures of attitude—arrogance, pride, and so on. It does not worry that hubristic activities actually endanger God. The sin is not in threatening God; the sin is of motivation. Futility, therefore, the pathetic waste of effort, is part and parcel of hubris. God is not actually in any danger from Eve or Babel's engineers, and their futile attempt to become Godlike is essentially a pointless misdirection of human energy and a waste of talent. When we rebel, we hurt ourselves, not God.[20]

To more directly apply this to RGTs, in what Hopkins perceives as the proper hubris objection, there is no danger of us becoming like God because of our reproductive technology abilities; God is beyond any threat from us. Mainline theologian Nancy Duff represents this perspective, saying in the context of debates about cloning that while issuing this warning against attempting to play God theologians should remind people that even the awesome ability to replicate humans would not actually turn us into gods. The belief that advances in scientific technology decrease the power of God as they proportionately increase human power itself represents hubris and self-deception. No matter how successful we are at putting together the right biological material to replicate life, we do not, as God does, call life into being.[21]

Critically, Hopkins writes that many religious elites in debates about RGTs are no longer using the classic notions of hubris, but are rather using a different conception of the relationship between God and humans—the Promethean. The story of Prometheus in the ancient Greek religion, for our purposes, is centered on the idea that Prometheus went to heaven and stole fire for humans from the gods who had been withholding it. The basic metaphor is that God has something, and humans steal it; thus, we are a threat to God. For example, an executive with the Southern Baptist Convention says that cloning "aims to usurp God's prerogatives as Creator," and a representative of the National Conference of Catholic Bishops says that cloning is an attempt to "exceed the limits of the delegated dominion given to the human race . . . [we are stealing something that belongs to God] . . . . that is, critics move from exposing the futility and arrogance of trying to do what only God can do to claiming that it is morally wrong to do what God can also do. . . . the hubris criticism is slowly changing into a Promethean criticism."[22] What this means is that "both believers and observers begin to think of humanity as a rival, competing with God over tangible powers. They begin to think of God as a kind of divine wizard whose magic spells are being deciphered or a divine programmer whose heavenly code is being hacked."[23]

Hopkins thinks that one of the problems with the Promethean notion of our relationship with God, compared to the hubris account, is that each bit of new understanding then steals something additional from God, thus further diminishing God. God becomes what Verhey has called a "God of the gaps," where God exists in the things that humans cannot explain or manipulate.[24]

What Hopkins gives us is a choice between a discourse of God that is Promethean, where certain actions are wrong because they usurp God prerogatives (e.g., stealing fire from Zeus), and a hubris discourse, where God cannot be stolen from, because no matter what, God is in control. In this latter discourse of God, the point is not "protecting God but about caring for the creation drawn from God."[25] We are not to draw lines around

God's technical abilities, but rather to fulfill God's desires for us. This makes the hubris position like the natural law position in that we are to follow what nature is supposed to be and can fix what is not supposed to be. With Promethean discourse, there are demarcated technical powers we are not supposed to have.

Closely related to the Promethean discourse is the idea that God has a plan for us genetically; therefore, it would be wrong to change it because part of God's powers is setting people's genetic futures. This is fatalism, a belief that there is a predetermined set of events that are and should be outside of human control.[26] In short, your genetic qualities are as they should be, because they were designed that way by God. Scholars have long studied how religiously inspired fatalism acts as a deterrent toward health behaviors, is associated with illness and disability, and leads to acquiescence in the face of disease.[27] Religiously inspired fatalism, where God's actions are outside of human control and what currently exists should not be interfered with, is what the Catholic natural law tradition is often mistaken for.

Religiously inspired fatalism has also long been a component of RGT debates among academics. For example, in the debates of the 1960s and 1970s, theologian Joseph Fletcher opposed other theologians for pronouncing that what God has created genetically must not be changed. Fletcher opposed "accidental or random reproduction," which he equated with a fatalistic response to one's genetic condition, and supported the antifatalistic approach of "rationally willed or chosen reproduction." He famously concluded "I cannot see how either humanity or morality are served by genetic roulette."[28]

If we return to the image of God promoted by the Promethean discourse, we see it is similar to the fatalistic view. The Promethean view suggests a God who is defined by powerful abilities, which are reserved only for God, such as the creation of life. The God of the fatalists not only has these powers but also expresses this capacity through their continuous use, deciding who is going to have which genetic trait. While these two discourses are intellectually distinct, they are so intertwined in the interviews with ordinary religious people that I will consider Promethean fatalism as one discourse.

Contemporary Bioethical Debate

When academic and activist *proponents* of RGTs describe the God they think opponents believe in, they describe a Promethean fatalist God that reserves certain powers or a hyper-Promethean fatalist God, where there are no powers allocated to humans, and any modification of nature is stealing from God. For example, James D. Watson, codiscoverer of the structure of DNA, wrote that "one of the greatest gifts science has brought to the world is continuing elimination of the supernatural," suggesting a God that can be diminished as we continue to steal fire through accumulated human knowledge.[29] Similarly, Lee Silver, a Princeton biologist and advocate of RGTs, says that "as is so often the case with new reproductive technologies, the real reason that people condemn cloning has nothing to do with technical feasibility, child psychology, societal well-being, or the preservation of the human species. The real reason derives from religious beliefs." Continuing, we can almost envision Prometheus sneaking behind Zeus's back to grab the fire when Silver says that religious people are opposed to cloning because "cloning leaves God out of the process of human creation and that man is venturing into places he does not belong."[30]

Or, consider philosopher John Harris, in the context of a discussion of improving humans through the insertion of animal genes into the human genome. He sees many people as objecting to this technology because it is "usurping God's prerogative and creating new life forms or perhaps disturbing the course of nature." We are, in Promethean terms, again stealing Zeus's fire. He continues by explaining the "playing God" objection to this technology:

> If it is supposed that we ought not to play God a number of assumptions must be made. The first is that God has a monopoly of the role; the second is that she is doing a good job (or a better one than we would do) and perhaps in consequence has a right to be left to get on with it; the third is perhaps that God's will is expressed in nature and that consequently the so-called natural order must not be disturbed. You don't have to be an atheist to see that the idea that we ought not to play God is a non-starter.[31]

Many bioethicists also have long described the God of religious opponents of RGTs as Promethean. For example, in a very influential text about human genetic engineering, a presidential bioethics commission in the early 1980s concluded that, when theologians use the term "playing God" in the context of human genetic engineering, what they mean is that it is not our role to interfere with the nature that God has created.[32]

By assuming that religious people use this Promethean fatalist discourse, these academics and advocates present hypothetical challenges to the believer who is opposed to RGTs. For example, Harris continues the passage above by describing a hyper-Promethean fatalist God who allocates no powers to humans, not even medical care, saying:

Even believers must believe it can be right to disturb and redirect the course of nature otherwise the practice of medicine itself would be wicked. For people naturally fall ill and naturally have reparable defects; if the practice of medicine has a coherent aim. It must be seen, if anything, as the comprehensive attempt to frustrate the course of nature. No one who believes it right to take an antibiotic or to vaccinate her children believes either that God is doing a great job unaided or that it is wrong to disturb the natural order. Moreover, the idea that human beings should not disturb what God has so carefully arranged presupposes that we and the disturbing things we do are not part of those arrangements.[33]

Or again, consider philosopher Gregory Pence. He argues that "the most general argument against creating an adult human being through [cloning] is that it is against the will of God. Some people believe that humans have no right to change the way that humans are created because sexual reproduction was ordained by God and that to try to change this way is sinful."[34] Sexual reproduction is the Promethean flame in this account, the power withheld from humans. He, like Harris, continues by arguing against a Promethean fatalist notion of God, which presumes that his interlocutor is a Promethean fatalist, and argues that the religious should use a "hubris" account of the relationship between God and humanity. Pence writes that one could argue that "because a rational God exists and cares about us, He allows us to make new discoveries in medicine and science" and "because God is rational and cares about us, he directs us to create humans in ways that are rational and that express caring about human beings."[35]

These two philosophers think that pointing out that religious people use medicine is devastating to religious opponents of RGTs, because they presume the religious use a Promethean fatalist discourse. Their interpretation of what this logically means is hyper-Promethean, where not even healthcare is a power allocated by God to humans. In fact, there are other discourses used by religious people, as we will see below, and nobody uses the hyper-Promethean discourse.

Secular Nature in the Religious Public

Most people with whom we spoke had a general preference for following nature, which, for many of the religious liberals, does not have any obvious religious referents. They have used this discourse in previous situations, such as preferring "natural" food, and are extremely ready to apply it to new situations, such as RGTs. The use of a secular discourse about following nature is not used to oppose RGTs that would alleviate what they consider to be a disease, but rather it is used by many of the (relative) supporters to oppose RGTs that they consider to be an enhancement, such as making children more intelligent.

This preference for the natural can be seen in our conversation with Shira, a middle-aged Reconstructionist Jew. Following our discussion of using preimplantation genetic diagnosis to make sure that a woman bore a girl or a boy, the interviewer asked her about using sperm sorting to accomplish the same end. She said that this was better because "it's not as technological. It's not as manipulative. I was going to say it's almost more natural, but it really isn't natural; it's just not as high-tech." Although she claims to see both as "not natural," clearly she uses the term "technology" as the inverse of natural; therefore, sperm sorting is "more natural." When she was asked why "not so high-tech" seemed better to her, she said that "as you get into this technology and all the potential and where it can go, and you get into those, you know, ethical issues being raised—the cloning and everything—I think the further removed you are from that, the more normal or regular or okay it seems—less technological and the more normal." She is basically saying the less technology is involved, the less need for ethical debates. Nature is given; it cannot be ethically controversial. Shira is assuming that what is natural is ideally the way it should be.

When the mainline Protestants, Jews, and secular people with whom we spoke wanted to oppose an RGT, they often invoked the discourse of safety that is also commonly used by bioethicists and scientists. This principle is quite simple: if a technology is not safe to its users, to others, or to the society, it should not be used. Many who use a discourse of safety simultaneously invoke a discourse that claims that "the natural" way is inherently more safe, because it has been "time-tested" in the words of one person with whom we spoke. Therefore, when connected to safety, we can derive the "ought" from "this is."

For example, among the people with whom we spoke who were forty years old or older, many remembered a margarine commercial that ran throughout the 1970s where a woman in a white gown is eating margarine and an off-screen narrator says, "That's Chiffon Margarine, not butter." When this woman, playing the role of Mother Nature, replies, "Margarine, oh, no, it's too sweet, too creamy," she becomes perturbed and produces lightening and thunder saying, "It's not *nice* to fool Mother Nature!"[36] People seem to remember this differently, saying that it is not nice to fool *with* Mother Nature.

For example, Francine is a self-identified liberal Protestant who attends her United Methodist congregation faithfully. She is concerned

> about consequences. I don't know that I have any religious views on it. I don't think there's anything that's based in my religion . . . I just feel we're so superficial as humans. We're just so stupid sometimes and . . . and I just feel that we don't always make wise choices and there are reasons after so many millions of years for humans to be the way they are and it's just . . . you know that old commercial about margarine: "Don't mess with Mother Nature." . . . We think we're awfully smart sometimes and we find down the line that we're not quite as smart as we thought we were.

Kay, another liberal Protestant, was supportive of most uses of RGTs. When it came to the few instances of enhancement RGTs to which she was opposed, she began, as many liberals did, by noting that "it's hard for me to tell other people what to do, but assuming that I were imposing my will," she would argue against, in this instance, preimplantation genetic diagnosis for sex selection:

> I don't think it's worth it just for the sake of making sure you have a girl. . . . I mean genetics can be a wonderful thing, but, you know, I just keep thinking of the old butter ad about "It's not nice to fool with Mother Nature," you know. . . . And because it's such a new thing, we may not yet know what all the repercussions are. I mean if they do this procedure to artificially make sure they have a girl, do we know for sure that that girl won't end up having some kind of problems later on as a result of this procedure? . . . And so, you know, if it's something where the child is going to live or die depending on if you do this, that's one thing, but whether it's a boy or girl, that seems—that, like the intelligence and the obesity, seems like a frivolous reason to be messing around with that kind of stuff . . . You know, the—the natural process, I think, is always the best choice.

It is also common to claim that the "natural way" is safer not only for the individual but also for the planet, because nature, it turns out, is inherently wise, having evolved into an equilibrium state that we should be cautious about changing. Many invoked analogies to global warming, which was seen as humans upsetting the delicate balance of nature. For example, Judy, a mainline Protestant, is supportive of most of the RGT applications that she considers to be promoting health. She says that when it comes to sex selection, "I think you need to leave that to nature, I just do." The reason is that "we've been here for a very long time without tampering with certain things and we've survived, and it happens every so often that's there's an outburst . . . a spurt of growth in more males one year but then it balances out the next year. So if Mother Nature has been doing okay on that end, why are we interfering?"

This secular sounding version of "following nature" is not the naturalistic fallacy because these people do not want to follow nature just because it is "nature." Rather, they are ultimately opposed for safety reasons, with the assumption that what is "natural" is safer. Presumably if some intervention could be shown to not be dangerous, these people would not use this discourse.

Natural Law

Others described the "natural" as created by God; therefore, God's authority over nature, as well as humans' relationship to God, becomes critical. As noted in the epigraph at the beginning of this chapter, following nature qua nature is usually expressed religiously. In the words of Jerry, a middle-aged evangelical who attends a Pentecostal church: "it's always kind of scary when society decides to embrace some technology . . . that would ultimately alter the natural design." When asked what he meant by "natural design," he said, "I think a lot of things that God has created to be is meant to be." Of those who spoke of a relationship between God and nature, there was a group of strong opponents who used the natural law discourse.

Many of the Catholics with whom we spoke, particularly those who identified themselves as traditionalist Catholics, articulated the natural law theory principle that the natural is "that which ought to be, not merely that which happens to be."[37] For example, Craig has an implicit theory of the natural human that ought to exist when he draws the line between acceptable and unacceptable applications of RGTs. He said, "God intended us to have hearing. God intended us to be able to breathe. God intended us to grow old, become wise and use our minds to teach others. On the other hand, whether or not we're all considered intelligent . . . Playing God, that's what it means to me." It is not "natural" for everyone to be intelligent, but it is for everyone to have hearing.

Theresa, who is opposed to all RGTs, has a different theory where the natural human is defined as the current genetic configuration of the species. After Theresa noted her opposition to all RGTs and applications of RGTs because they are "interfering with God's plan," the interviewer asked, "But, aren't we interfering with God's natural processes or whatever when we give penicillin to somebody with pneumonia?" "No, we are not," she replied, because "you're not ultimately changing them. It's not at the basic foundation of life. You're not changing them as a fundamental being." Another Catholic woman approved of RGTs to treat diseases. When asked why she would not approve of using RGTs to improve intelligence, she said that "seems to me to be more of a natural kind of a thing, like the color of my eyes." Eye color and intelligence are natural, part of the way God wanted us to be. Diseases are implicitly not natural, not part of the normative human, and can therefore be ameliorated.

The Hubris Discourse

The hubris discourse was commonly used by the (relative) proponents to justify their conclusions for the technologies that they supported (typically for disease) in contrast to those that they opposed (typically for enhancement). There were a number of ways the respondents use the hubris discourse, where no technology is inherently reserved for God. The most prominent is to say that God gave us brains in order to do God's work on this earth, so God is working through humans. The image is that God *wants* us to develop the "magical" abilities that the Promethean account attributes to God. Consider Beatrice, a traditional evangelical, who says that there is no technology *itself* that is stealing something from God:

> It goes back to the sense that God has given us these abilities and this intelligence to create penicillin to wipe out, not wipe out, but to able to fight bacterial diseases, to create drugs that combat cancer and other disease. It gives me medicine to take for my thyroid to make it work right, and I think that is all good stuff. I think there can be good stuff coming out of genetics and genetic

technology. But there is always the flip side of how that technology is going to be used. I mean, we create all these drugs, and we also create dangerous viruses that can be used as weapons. That is the flip side of everything. God has given us the ability, so I can't. . . . I don't believe you can say, "Okay, God alone can do this," but on the other hand I believe you have to be willing to look at things as not just as "What can I do?" but "What should I do? What is the right thing to do?" Unfortunately, too many people don't care about what is right. They just want to do whatever they want to do because they can do it. I think that is a problem.

Alice, another traditional evangelical, explained her similar view through a story that anyone who has spent a lifetime in a church would eventually hear:

> There was a man in his house during a torrential rain, and the firemen came by and told him to leave for his own safety. And the man says, "No, I have faith in God." And so he goes up on the roof as the water rises and the police come and ask him to leave and everything. And the man says, "No, I have faith in God, God will save me." Then a sailboat came by. They tell him to step in the boat, you know that it's flooded, you know, everybody's evacuated and he says, "No, I have faith in God, I'm staying and I'm not leaving my house." . . . Pretty soon the helicopter comes and they let down a rope for him to grab on, you know, that if he doesn't get off that roof soon the house is just gonna wash away and he's gonna die. He says, "No, I have faith in God. God's gonna take care of me and I'm gonna stay right here." So the man dies and he gets to Heaven and he asks the Lord, "You know, I had faith in You and—and You didn't save me. Why didn't You save me?" And He said, "I sent the firemen. I sent the helicopters. . . . " You know, so it's kind of like that, you know. I mean, His hands are our hands, you know. And so if He has sent things that we can use to help us then, yeah. Go for it.

A related theme is expressed by Jack, a middle-aged fundamentalist who has a more interventionist God in mind. It is not so much that God gave us the brains to figure things out, but rather that God allows us in each instance to develop a technology. He told us that "certainly we've been given technology by God to use. A lot of times it gets misused but I believe the technology is there because God allows us to have it. Why? I don't know exactly and why did he wait so long to decide to give us some of the technology that we do have? I don't know. . . . I mean, using the analogy that I've used, it's just like a medical procedure that would eradicate any other kind of disease." A young mainline Protestant woman said something similar when asked whether the ability to change the genes of the human species should be reserved for God. "God has given us the ability to do it," she began; "So, apparently, God doesn't think it should be reserved for God 'cause He's already letting us do it."

Another way of expressing the hubris discourse is to say that God gave us free will that we can use for good or evil. Jim is a moderate Catholic who works for the military. When asked whether God wants us to create these new technologies, he told us:

> Sure. . . . I think he's just sitting up there kind of like a father watching us play in the sandbox with our little toys and tools and just kind of awed by it, you know? "Look at them go." . . . We should exercise our own free will. Sure. I'm sure we create technologies, you know, the atom bomb or things of that nature as appalling as it is, He probably kind of cringed here and there but then again, you know, he's not going to stop us. What's interesting is that, you know, there he is. He's kind of like a father. He's like "okay, pal. You want to go do that? You're going to live with the consequences." You go out and have a few beers and crash your car. "Told you so." So it's like "you're going to create these nuclear bombs, you're going to use them. Okay, fine. Go ahead. See what's going to happen." Whoosh.

In this imagery, humans are on their own to invent or not to invent RGTs, but certain choices would violate God's desires for us. Alice emphasized another similar theme, that is, the technologies themselves are not good or bad, but it is only their uses that can result in sin:

> God gives us choice, doesn't He? Does He want us to sin? Does He want us to blow up people with a time bomb? Does He want us to kill people with guns? He gave people the knowledge to be able to create those things, then guns are not necessarily bad, are they? It is, they're used to kill, food, game that we need to eat, right? Okay. But then they can be bad 'cause they can be used to kill man. So, the same way with those technologies, again what we use them for? And what our intent, motives are—how far you go with it.

Another moderate Catholic, when asked if God wants us to create these new technologies, said that she did not "think God has an opinion on that. I don't think He cares one way or the other." She continued by saying:

I'm a free willer. God might be disappointed if we make a mistake and He might be excited if we improve our lot of life but you know, God has stood by for a lot of mistakes and hasn't taken his ball and gone home yet. So this is irrelevant to him. You know what I'm saying? It's just a small thing to God. "Let them mess around with it if they want to and you know, maybe they'll do some good. They've done some good in the past and maybe they won't. I might step in" and like he said in the Bible, "I might step in if they're making a huge mistake and I might not."

Promethean Fatalist Discourse

There *was* a strong minority of the in-depth interviewees who used the Promethean fatalistic discourse of the relationship between humans and God, and these interviewees were the strongest opponents of RGTs. Importantly, while the religious citizens in general are more opposed to RGTs than the nonreligious, the survey shows that if the respondent uses the Promethean fatalistic discourse concerning the relationship between God and humans to describe RGTs in general, they are more opposed to RGTs.[38] We can then say that the disproportionate use of Promethean fatalism is a reason that religious people tend to be more opposed to RGTs than the nonreligious. Since these people are opposed to the most RGTs and their applications, I will more closely examine the use of this discourse for different RGTs and its relationship to the abortion issue.

I provide separate descriptions of the use of Promethean fatalism for pro-lifers and non–pro-lifers—those who do and do not use the embryonic life discourse. If the pro-lifers use the Promethean fatalist discourse to oppose abortion as well as the other RGTs, then the issues will be merged, and existing theories would predict that others would not want to discuss RGTs with the pro-lifers because it will be perceived to be as pointless as deliberating abortion. However, if the pro-lifers and at least some of the non–pro-lifers both use the Promethean fatalist discourse for the same or similar issues, then there is no communicative barrier for these groups and the forces discouraging future deliberation will be mitigated.

Promethean Fatalist Pro-lifers

In the survey reported in table 3 in chapter 3, 92 percent of the pro-lifers who are strong opponents of RGTs also use the Promethean fatalist discourse. While this is suggestive, it cannot tell us *which* RGTs they would use this for, nor whether they would use it if not asked by the survey. In the in-depth interviews, if this type of person is asked what they think about abortion for cystic fibrosis, they will typically use both discourses. For example, José, when discussing amniocentesis, starts by using the embryonic life discourse, saying:

> I don't believe in abortion. You know, some people talk that way, what if it was rape or there's incest. A life is a life. That child had nothing to do with the situation and I don't believe in abortion under any circumstances. . . . If I knew it wouldn't lead to an abortion, I'd say yes, go ahead and have it tested. Otherwise, if they're kind of lingering on the margin, I'd say . . . I guess I'd trust in God, in all things.

In other words, you should trust that God has a plan for you that you should not modify.

When we next talked about preimplantation genetic diagnosis for cystic fibrosis, José was opposed to that as well, but shifted away from the embryonic life discourse:

> It's science playing God, and it always goes back to that trust. Even if the cows should die or something, we always make it through our situations. Because [me and my spouse] had a [very difficult personal situation], and it was a very rough situation, but we made it through it, and I think anybody can do it. I do. I think if they have that trust there isn't anything you can't overcome. I think that's wrong, ethically wrong, in my opinion.[39]

He continued:

> I'm a true believer that God has a plan for each one of us. We can either learn that plan through the divine—Him leading us, letting God lead us—or we can go our own way. So if there's a child that has . . . that would be born with cystic fibrosis and this child somehow has a key to discovering the cause or prevention of cystic fibrosis, if they were to abort that child, they'll never have that key. I believe science is going a little too far as far as changing, splicing genes, whatever you want to call it. And our world has gone too far in trusting in man rather than trusting in God.

The difficult personal situation to which he refers is, for him, analogous to preimplantation genetic diagnosis for cystic fibrosis, and in both situations you are to trust that God has a plan you are not to intervene in. For sperm sorting for sex, which does not implicate embryos, he continued using the Promethean fatalist discourse:

> Again, for me it goes back to that . . . well, you know, I thought . . . I always wanted a big family. God's going to give me so many boys and so many girls, okay. It's his plan for me. So if I go and say I want all boys and start messing with things, that to me is taking that out of God's hands and saying to the doctor, you be God now. This is what I want you to do for me. Instead of asking, okay, you gave me a daughter. I wanted a boy but you gave me a daughter. Why did you do that or what do you want me to do now? We took things as they came, we knew that . . . we had [one child] when we were [older],[40] and we knew that the older my wife got that Down's syndrome was a possibility and we talked about it. And we both decided, hey, if that's what happens, that's our child, it will not be treated any differently other than special needs and we'll love it just as much as we do the other seven. I have a very big issue with science sorting eggs or things like that.

He uses the same Promethean fatalist discourse he used to discuss abortion, but in a situation where no embryos are threatened. This suggests that José views sperm sorting as part of a broader issue that includes abortion because both fit the same previous situation of his earlier family planning decisions.

Like others who also used the embryonic life and Promethean fatalist discourses, José did *not* use the Promethean fatalist discourse to talk about human genetic engineering for cystic fibrosis. To reiterate, we portrayed this as not involving the destruction of embryos, and the embryonic life discourse then does not appear to fit. Although you would think it would also be analogous to sperm sorting for sex, where he would take what God gives him, instead there was a more salient feature of the new situation. He responded:

> That to me is a cure, okay? And there's nothing wrong with curing disease, because it's done pre-conception I guess. You're not messing with, you're not really messing with the act of conception. That way I think, just like curing smallpox or something like that. You want to wipe those things out, yeah. If you could find a cure for . . . like we did polio, because I don't know if that was a genetic thing or a virus thing I'm not sure. But for stuff like that if you can find a cure and give a shot to cure any gene that I have in my body that has a chance

of making a child of mine perfect. That's okay because it's not dealing with . . . to me, it's not dealing with the act of conception. Yeah, if you can give a shot for those things. That's just like flu shots, stuff like that. You're helping people that way. Once you get into the decision making of whether that's going to be a boy or a girl, stuff like that, that's where I have to draw the line I think. But yeah. You want a cure for diseases I think everybody does. I don't want decision making for me, as in, you have a cystic fibrosis gene but we can mess around with this stuff here, separate all these things and fix it that way. To me, that's not in God's plan. I'm not saying that science is bad. Science is there to help men, but it's not there to take over the job of decision-making for God. That's the way I look at it.

Why does he not use the Promethean fatalist discourse to oppose human genetic engineering for cystic fibrosis? We might think that it is part of God's plan for a child and all of that child's descendants to have cystic fibrosis. The answer is that for most of the people who use the Promethean fatalist discourse, the specific application of human genetic engineering for cystic fibrosis does not have an analogy with abortion, but with medical care. That they cannot use the same discourses—even if we might think they would be able to—means that human genetic engineering for health reasons is not similar to the other RGTs and is unlikely to be considered part of the abortion issue.

When the conversation moves to human genetic engineering for conditions that are not as grave as cystic fibrosis, he uses the Promethean fatalist discourse again. When asked about its use for early onset Alzheimer's, he does not answer directly, but describes the situations where he uses the Promethean fatalist discourse:

I think any cure for any ailment is fine as long as it doesn't conflict with creation of life in God's plan, I guess. The way He meant things to be. To me, there's a reason for our friends having a Down's syndrome baby. I don't know why that is but there's a reason. And there's a reason for [what happened to our child.] I don't know what that is but I think God had a reason. So I accept things like that.[41]

Avoiding Down's syndrome is not like avoiding cystic fibrosis for José, but Down's syndrome is part of God's plan that should not be interfered with. Also in God's realm is using human genetic engineering to modify intelligence, about which he said:

I think God put variety in life, so to speak. I know I'm not as smart as this doctor, but I'm not as unintelligent as another man down the road. I think He's
given us all our spots and our lives and our plans that we should try to live out
the life that He wants us to live. . . . No, I don't think they should be playing with
that either.

In response to whether a couple should clone a friend of theirs that they
admire, he responds, "No. Definitely not. . . . to me, it takes three to make
a baby. A husband and wife. Not a husband, a wife and some friend. It
takes a husband, a wife, and God to create that child."

In sum, Joe uses the Promethean fatalist discourse with the embryonic
life discourse, and when embryonic life no longer fits, he continues to use
the Promethean fatalist. The exception is human genetic engineering for
cystic fibrosis, a situation that has some feature that makes it appear to be
medical care and not like previous situations for which the Promethean
fatalist discourse has been used.

Similarly, we spoke with Patricia, a Catholic stay-at-home mom who is
opposed to amniocentesis. She started by talking about what she saw as
the inaccuracy of the amniocentesis test. She said that people should "just
wait because the test may mean other things. I've known people who've
had false positives for certain tests, and the stress that they put on themselves during the rest of the pregnancy worrying about it is more harmful
than the outcome." Later, she continued using discourses that I will examine in later chapters:

> I—I just believe that not everybody is perfect, you know, and—you know [I
> don't agree] that they should be . . . aborting babies because they think some-
> thing's wrong with it. Because then in essence, you know, they're saying that
> down the line they want to have children [that are]—in the entire world being
> normal or perfect. And I don't know that I necessarily agree with that.

When we talked about preimplantation genetic diagnosis for cystic fibrosis, she combined the embryonic life and Promethean fatalist discourses,
saying:

> That sounds good, but I still think that once those eggs are fertilized, then
> they're basically aborting it. Where if it's fertilized, then that's the start of a
> new life. So if they're testing it and they find out that it has cystic fibrosis, then
> they're just going to discard it. And I don't agree with that. I don't agree with

abortion and things like that. I feel that, you know, God, you know, gives us the miracle of life, and I don't think it's up to us to decide when to discard it.

Shortly thereafter, the conversation turned to using preimplantation genetic diagnosis to determine the sex of a child, and while she could also have used the embryonic life discourse here, she used the Promethean fatalist discourse:

> I think that if you truly want children, you know . . . truly you'll love them— you'll love them whether it's a boy or a girl. . . . But I don't think that it's—again, I guess it's—my religious beliefs are coming into play here. You know, God gives you what He thinks you can handle. And [if you decide] whether you want a girl or boy, then you don't truly want a child as bad as you think you do.

God gives you what you can handle—that is, sex selection is interfering with God's plan for you. She reiterates this claim with sperm sorting, concluding that "God gives you what He knows you can handle," showing that this discourse used in the abortion debate can be used for applications that have nothing to do with embryos.

When the conversation turns to human genetic engineering for cystic fibrosis, she, like others, keeps pushing this toward a distinct issue domain until she approves of it. We started with our standard description of Sam and Sue who "have two children and both of their children have cystic fibrosis. And let's say that the doctor perfected a new technique where now not only could he test the fertilized egg, but he can actually change the gene in the fertilized egg to remove any chance that the baby . . . would have cystic fibrosis. So if Sam and Sue had a baby in this way . . . not only would that baby be free of cystic fibrosis, the baby's children and grandchildren and forever down the line of that family tree would all be free of cystic fibrosis. So do you think that they should do this?" One might think that the part of the scenario that describes changing the genes of an entire family into the future might be salient for her, and be analogous to situations where Promethean fatalism has been previously used, but like other respondents, that was not the case.

Patricia responded: "So they can only do it to the fertilized egg. They couldn't do it for the parents—remove the gene from the parent before they got pregnant?" The interviewer asked if that sounded better to her, and since it did, the interview continued about that imagined technology, with a shot. With our original scenario, Patricia does not like the idea that if modification of the embryo went wrong, it would be destroyed, saying, "I guess maybe if they can test it and remove it and . . . then if it didn't work—you know, take, or what-have-you, the person's still going to have the baby no matter what, then that might be an option that, to me, doesn't sound that bad."

This is not a surprising position to take for someone who uses the embryonic life discourse—she is essentially concerned about an accident with the human genetic engineering technology as we originally described it. What is important is that with her preferred technology, where the parents' genes are changed before they try to have children (thus changing the genes of their offspring), "sound[s] better to me because then the whole process of the pregnancy and everything is more natural." In response to the question "Why natural?" she responded:

> It's more of God's will and God's doing if it's all natural and not technology coming into play. . . . I agree with—you know, people that are sick, they find cures and things like that for—[but] that's natural or, you know, more of a God-given thing, not actually going and alter the genetics of these embryos and things like that.

This is a bit unclear, but when we get to the next question about human genetic engineering for Alzheimer's disease, she becomes more clear. "I look upon that being as natural, as more of a cure, which is what I'm more for, rather than actually alteration of the things. So, no. I mean if it's the shot and it's going to be natural, I'm more okay with that than trying to alter the embryo—you know, the fetus itself." As long as she can be assured that embryos or fetuses will not be hurt, she approves of what she considers to be health applications of human genetic engineering.

What is important is that Patricia argues that we can modify a person's existing body to remove a gene, with that change being inherited by the children, even if it has the same result as modifying an embryo. Even in her modified scenario of modifying an existing body, Promethean fatalism does not fit, even though her modified scenario is also, we would think, "playing God" with future generations of humans. Modifying future generations or intervening in God's realm does not seem to be the salient feature of this new situation, but rather healing across generations is; thus, the respondents draw analogies to other cases of intergenerational healing (e.g., "finding cures").

By the time the interview gets to other enhancements that do not harm embryos, Patricia returns to the Promethean fatalist discourse. In discussing cloning, which she thinks is "actually kind of gross," she makes an argument about the need for people to be individuals, and then reiterates what she said before that we should just accept what God offers to us:

> Again, I don't think you should—if you truly want a child, you'll love what you have. And if you're going to pick and choose, it's like going to the grocery store and picking out what you like to eat, and doing that for a child, then can you truly love that child [if] he wasn't—you know, just a normal, regular person?

Both José and Patricia opposed most RGTs, but approved of human genetic engineering for cystic fibrosis. This was a pattern in the in-depth interview data, but not in the survey. What is important for my argument is not the number of people who opposed human genetic engineering for cystic fibrosis in either data source, but that they did not use Promethean fatalism to do so, because human genetic engineering for cystic fibrosis is then for them in a distinct domain.

For example, Steve had just said that he was opposed to sperm sorting because "I don't believe in trying to help God make this baby for us. . . . Maybe God doesn't intend for us to have it. I think He intends for us to have what we have." In the next discussion, he is opposed to human genetic engineering for cystic fibrosis, but, using a "safety" discourse, says: "That's pretty deep stuff, messing with genes. Right off, I would say no. I would say no, leave it alone [because] it may go away. It may not be in this family tree. Things leave and other things come in. Maybe something would come in worse than that." For Steve, human genetic engineering for cystic fibrosis clearly is not an analogous situation to abortion, sperm sorting, or other RGTs; therefore, for Steve and people like him, human genetic engineering for cystic fibrosis is unlikely to be incorporated into an opposition to genetic control issue domain because different discourses are used.

Promethean Fatalist Non–pro-lifers

Many of the non–pro-lifers—those who do not use the embryonic life discourse—use the hubris and secular nature discourses, but many use the Promethean fatalist discourse to state their opposition to at least some RGTs as do the pro-life strong opponents. I separately examine two groups of people on this side of the supposed discursive boundary (fig. 3, *right*) because they provide distinct descriptions of the discursive divide between the two supposed sides of the culture war: a very porous and moderately porous divide.

The first group is identical to the pro-life strong opponents we just discussed in that they reach the same conclusions about the same RGTs and use the same discourses—except the embryonic life discourse that divides the two sides of the culture war. These people then have an extremely porous divide with those on the other side of the embryonic life divide because they share so many discourses for so many applications of RGTs.

However, they are not the dominant group among the non–pro-lifers who use the Promethean fatalist discourse. The larger group is the (relative) proponents who reach the same conclusions as the strong opponents only for enhancements, but *do* use the same discourse as the strong opponents. (Since this is the larger group, they are portrayed in fig. 3.) These people have a moderately porous divide where shared conclusions and discourses exist on some issues that could be the basis of a conversation on remaining issues of disagreement.

Rudy is a Catholic who is opposed to amniocentesis and is one of those who has an extremely porous divide. While opposed to abortion for cystic fibrosis like those on the other side of the divide, he does not use the embryonic life discourse, but rather uses the other three oppositional discourses examined in this book to make his case. As Rudy explained:

> And this is just a personal thing, I wouldn't test it at all. That's our baby; we're going to have it. We'll just make it work. Whatever happens, happens. If God decides that we're the one in four [whose child has cystic fibrosis] then we are. If we're not, then we thank him. We're going to move in a totally different direction. But no, I wouldn't test it at all. I don't believe I'd ever have an abortion or ask my wife to do that. No. It would be a done deal. We'd move on and make it work.

With preimplantation genetic diagnosis for cystic fibrosis, which for pro-lifers is often the occasion to talk about embryos, Rudy simply reiterates his Promethean fatalism to justify his opposition:

> No. No. I guess I'm from the old school and I think everything is meant to be for a reason. I don't think that when you start messing with science and dealing with the things that are really out of your control. I guess I never have believed in that. My [children] were born and I had no idea they were going to [have a particular cosmetic trait.] . . . I think it's a gift no matter what you get.[42]

When presented with the scenario of sperm sorting, which does not involve any embryos, Rudy says that they should not do that "for the same reasons I said earlier." As in the situation from his own life described in the extract above, he thinks they should just have a child and "let's see what it's going to be."

When the conversation turns to human genetic engineering for cystic fibrosis—to "fix the genes in fertilized eggs to remove the chance that any baby would have cystic fibrosis"—Rudy turns supportive and does not use the Promethean fatalist discourse. He says, "I don't think I would have a problem with that. I think that's a little bit of a different scenario." He then goes on to approve of human genetic engineering for what he considers to be health conditions, like deafness and obesity, before opposing human genetic engineering for intelligence. He does not see the use of this technology for "health" reasons as similar to the other RGTs, but rather as a sort of medical treatment, showing us the limits of the Promethean fatalist discourse.

For the final type of enhancement we asked about, cloning, Rudy says, "Now that one really bothers me a lot. . . . To me, that goes back to that same thing. It's people wanting to know what they're going to have and get before it happens. If we can manipulate it a certain way it works the way we like it, let's go ahead and manipulate that." With cloning, as with most other RGTs, God will give us what we are supposed to have.

More common are non–pro-lifers who are (relative) supporters only opposed to enhancements. Their use of the Promethean fatalist discourse to oppose enhancements is otherwise the same as the pro-lifers who oppose most RGTs. This indicates a moderately porous boundary with those on the other side of the supposed communicative divide, as the discourse is shared for a number of applications of RGTs. Consider Jody, a nontraditional evangelical. When simply asked what a couple should do if they both had the genes for cystic fibrosis, she goes back and forth, without necessarily making a solid conclusion:

> But, you know, there's also that joy of having kids and raising them and the fact that just because the child has cystic fibrosis, doesn't mean that they can't, you know, be a blessing to the world or might bring something into the world that, you know, needs to be here. It's kind of a complicated question. (Laughs) What should they do? I don't know. It's so hard.

She invokes the Promethean fatalist discourse when she says, "It's like, I would pray a lot and try to sort it out that way. [*laughs*] I don't know. I guess a lot of that I think should be left up to faith, like maybe I wasn't supposed to have a kid, you know."

She is ambivalent about amniocentesis, because the test occurs so far into pregnancy and she clearly has an implicit developmental notion of when the fetus becomes a person. By the time the interview gets to preimplantation genetic diagnosis for cystic fibrosis, she is also torn:

> Wow. I haven't heard that. Oh, that's so hard. Because in a way it seems like you're, I would say, playing God. . . . I just worry about the other embryos. But, since you're having babies naturally, there would be only one that would fertilize anyway, so . . . I mean, unless, you had two at one time or whatever.

We can see that Jody does not have the orthodox version of the embryonic life discourse in that she considers it important that when people try to have babies "naturally," many eggs do not fertilize. In her agonizing, she uses the Promethean fatalist discourse, saying:

> I know from a logical perspective if you are presented with this possibility of having a child that's not going to have cystic fibrosis . . . I mean I don't know. It just seems to take out a lot of room for God to work in the situation. Again, I know, it's so funny. It's like I have these two sides in myself that fight. I have the science side and then the religion side and they can coincide.

She does not elaborate further on the idea of giving room to God to work. Ultimately, she does not use the Promethean fatalist discourse, concluding that, for this technology:

> I would think it's certainly a viable option. . . . If I was Bob and Barbara, I would say they would certainly have the right to do that. I certainly think that there should be no law that would prevent them from using that and they could certainly do that. For us, I'd have to think about it if it was us because you've got those other five that are sitting there. We would probably consider it though, for sure, seriously, if it was us.

While not using the embryonic life discourse, she clearly thinks that embryonic destruction is a serious matter. Preimplantation genetic diagnosis should certainly be available, and she would consider it for herself, but was not sure in the end whether she would use it.

For preimplantation genetic diagnosis for early onset Alzheimer's, Jody concludes that this would also be okay, because it is a disease. "If I think it's viable for the people that have cystic fibrosis in their family, I think if it's viable for one genetic disorder, I don't see why it wouldn't be viable for others. If people decided to make the choice that it was okay to do it for one, then it should be okay for all of them." Genetic characteristics that are all considered by this respondent to be "diseases" are all considered to be the same, the Promethean fatalist discourse is not used, and these diseases are thus in the same domain that I am calling "health promotion" (See fig. 3).

Jody equivocates with preimplantation genetic diagnosis for deafness, debating with herself whether deafness is a disease. She jumps off of the slippery slope at preimplantation genetic diagnosis for obesity:

> No, no. That's not . . . I think no. This is where it's starting to get, like I say with the physical appearance, I think then they're going to want to control the eye color and all of this kind of thing. I don't know why I consider that to be the line. I'm sure it's in different places for different people. But, for me, you take a little bit of the surprise out of it. [laughs] Have some fun and let go a little bit. That's another way from the spiritual perspective, let God have some room to work. The person might have this gene, but maybe they won't.

At the jumping off point, we are to leave room for God to work and ultimately it is up to God. Harris could of course argue that she is not being consistent, but actually she is using this discourse similarly to how others use it because disease is not what is to be left to God. She just has a different notion of what is God's responsibility than portrayed by the academic writers. As we would expect, she was supportive of human genetic engineering for cystic fibrosis—it was like chemotherapy she thought—and was opposed to applications of human genetic engineering that she thought were enhancements.

Maureen, a nontraditional evangelical, is similar. She was opposed to amniocentesis for opaque reasons. She then approves of preimplantation genetic diagnosis for cystic fibrosis:

> I would say that'd be worth further investigation. You know I would be comfortable with that. We certainly know people who have had children using the in-vitro fertilization, that's been a good solution . . . and providing there's no risk to the baby and that type of thing. Obviously when you're using that type of technique, you know, you're choosing which one to implant and which ones not to anyway so that's just a way of selecting which one's you're going to be using. That would be something I would consider.

Her next statement makes it clear why she was opposed to amniocentesis but not pre-implantation genetic diagnosis. When asked whether preimplantation genetic diagnosis is better than amniocentesis, she states that it is, because "to me it's because before it actually is a viable fetus in the womb that could have a chance of surviving." She has, like many Americans, a perspective where the fetus becomes a person much later in pregnancy, and is clearly not using the embryonic life discourse. She subsequently opposes preimplantation genetic diagnosis for early onset Alzheimer's, invoking a distinction in levels of suffering I will describe in subsequent chapters.

Later, she describes the boundary between domains for us, that society should allow technologies "based on only those that are life threatening [and those] that are more critical. In other words you get to the point where people start picking for intelligence and appearance and heights and all these other types of things that I think . . . only if it would be life threatening." "Why that line," she was asked. She responded:

> I would say that that's basically part of the complicated nature of what comes together of putting together a person and that there's not necessarily good or bad combinations, just different and we have to look at there's basically a creator that basically puts people together in a certain way for a certain reason and that whole idea of genetic selection would be limited for extreme purposes when it's only life threatening for the child.

She is basically saying we should stick to God's plan, except in cases of extreme suffering, a typical weighing for the Promethean non–pro-lifers. This use shows the actual meaning of the Promethean fatalist discourse— God has given us powers over medical care already, but not genetic enhancement. By the time we get to preimplantation genetic diagnosis for sex, she reiterates the point:

MAUREEN: Um, to me that's just too much control. I think there has to be some element of the divine plan as far as what your family is and what you desire to have. You know you can't want to have that but often times in hindsight you can realize why that was the right combination or why it worked out well for your family and so I would just say no. I really wouldn't select on some subjective criteria like that.

INTERVIEWER: Can you tell me a little bit about what you mean by the divine plan for your family?

MAUREEN: Well I'm just saying that there are certain things . . . if we knew everything in advance we probably wouldn't you know, get out of bed in the morning . . . I think one has to have a little bit of a faith based approach to life and
realize that the things that happen to you with the kind of family you have are
really part of an overall plan for your life that God has already prepared for you
and that is something is a part of but there's not a good or bad or right or wrong,
it's just really a matter of how you respond to it. So that type of control would be
like to me . . . you know just taking a little too much into your own hands.

With the logic of her moral line described for us, she continues feeling
for the boundary between the genetic enhancement and health promotion
domains. Human genetic engineering for cystic fibrosis is "just preven-
tative medicine." With human genetic engineering for obesity, "if we're
talking about . . . some sort of family history of morbid obesity, that is
something that is very serious, then yes of course. But if someone's just
saying I just want thin children, I think that's a little bit too much." With
human genetic engineering for intelligence she again feels for her line
by saying "I think that's a little bit much but . . . If you're talking about
something that's a gene that prevents some sort of low intelligence . . . that
prevents mental retardation or prevents something like that, that's different other than saying you're going to give them more and more and more
intelligence. Well, where do you draw the line?"

We also spoke with Colleen, an older Pentecostal woman. She starts by
laying out an argument about abortion that does not use the embryonic
life discourse:

I'm a believer and I'm not real big on abortion, unless it is because of health
reasons to that baby or the mother. But it's knowing, you know, God. I believe
he does form the children in the womb and life when they are first conceived
so he knows all things and if they are willing to trust the Lord to give them
whatever He feels they may need. But if they really have an issue in their heart,
"well I can't stand to have a child to have that or to know that I carry the gene
that made my child have it or I just really don't want children," then they need
to really seriously think that through.

Again, we could consider this to be inconsistent in that she is invoking
the Promethean fatalist discourse about God having a plan for you in the
womb, but also arguing that in some instances people can have an abortion anyway. This is because the actual meaning of Promethean fatalism

for those in this group means that it is not used in situations that are perceived to be improving health.

She approves of preimplantation genetic diagnosis for cystic fibrosis, but opposes preimplantation genetic diagnosis for deafness. When we discuss sex selection, she uses the Promethean fatalist discourse again, equating it to previous situations where you should trust God:

> I don't know. You know, I certainly wouldn't condemn them for doing it. I just kind of take what the Lord gives you. . . . I don't know. . . . So when you go to start picking out I want a boy or I want a girl is then like you become God and how do you know who is going to be an asset in our family? I don't know. Then I'm not really for genetically picking the genders.

When we return to what she considers to be diseases, with our discussion of human genetic engineering for cystic fibrosis, she is in favor again. She warns us that because of the fallen nature of humanity, we cannot make

> people perfect, but there is always going to be something because we are fallen, we are just a fallen generation. If it's not going to be cystic fibrosis, it's going to be, you know, HIV out here. There will always be something but if we could remove the cystic fibrosis, I think that, to me, would be okay.

She shows us how she sorts different applications of human genetic engineering into different domains through the use of the Promethean fatalist discourse: "But then I'm not of the thought where you need to plant this gene here and that gene there, make a high IQ or a blond-haired or a female or male, then that's God's business." Again, while this is "God's business," it is our business to heal what she considers to be disease. Cloning is "just ridiculous," she continues, because "that's God's business to create that baby. Then you are putting creating the baby in human hands and we are fallible people. It will become competitive. It will be high dollar. If you have more money, you'll get the better baby. You'll get the more with the genes. Society commercializes and will take over and God does not work that way. He is the creator of life."

Finally, consider our conversation with Coretta, an African American Catholic woman who is in favor of most of the applications of all the RGTs. She is not bothered by the destruction of embryos in amniocentesis or preimplantation genetic diagnosis. The salient feature for Coretta for most of the applications is disease, so she has a much more expansive

health promotion issue domain than most respondents because her definition of health is very broad. She only draws the line at intelligence, which
is a very strong line to her. Parents who try to use preimplantation genetic
diagnosis to select the most intelligent embryo are "trying to play God.
You can't do that. No one's perfect but God." When asked what "playing
God" means, she said, "Playing God is trying to do things that God would
do. We don't have control of certain things. No matter how much science
work you do, certain things we just don't have control over. That's for God
to do. We need to leave that alone." She also uses the Promethean fatalist
discourse to oppose human genetic engineering for intelligence:

> It gets me because, to me, you're playing God again. You're trying to do things
> that He has control of and I don't think no man has control of what God has. If
> God wanted you like that, then it would've been like that. Just sad things hap-
> pen to people. Don't get me wrong, I mean there is sad, but I really think if it
> was to be like God wanted it to be, you're just playing God. You don't need to
> be God. Just let God do His thing, and keep your faith, and pray, and let man
> just do the mediocre thing.

Cloning produces the same argument. "I'm not for that," she begins.
"That's once again playing God. That's, to me, ridiculous and they have
tried it. I don't agree with that. God gave women certain things and men
certain things and that's the way it should be. You have choices to do certain things. Like I say, if it's positive, go for it. But all this other stuff, talking about you gonna do, no. No, I don't want no one looking like me in
the whole world, other than if I have a twin. And God did that, not man.
Okay? I'm not for this cloning."

If we look at the non–pro-lifers who use the Promethean fatalist discourse, the discourse for some is used to oppose abortion for cystic fibrosis
and all applications of preimplantation genetic diagnosis, as well as for
enhancements that do not endanger embryos. For others, the Promethean
fatalist discourse is only used to oppose enhancements. This demonstrates
that the hyper-Promethean fatalist imagery used by academics is not
found among ordinary people—nobody thinks that God wants to keep
the power of improving health from humans. Of course, people differ in
what they see as the salient feature of new RGT situations, with some
focusing on the "health" aspect, and others seeing a situation that is analogous to previous situations where we should trust God. But, everyone has
at least one RGT that they perceive as being about health.

People on both sides of the supposed communication divide of the abortion debate use the Promethean fatalism discourse, with those with a more porous divide using the discourse to oppose the same RGTs as the strong opponents on the other side of the divide, and those with the moderately porous divide using the discourse to oppose only enhancements. Returning to the survey, we find that 74 percent of the non–pro-lifer (relative) proponents of RGTs do use Promethean fatalism to oppose at least some RGTs.[43] This suggests almost no discursive divide between the two sides because people on both sides use this discourse at some point, but the in-depth interviews suggest that there is a moderately porous divide as the two sides largely use the discourses for somewhat different sets of issues.

The Social Location of Promethean Fatalism

Discourses are available to people differentially according to their social location. For example, people in different eras only have access to particular discourses, such as the positive discourse about homosexuality that has only become available in certain parts of the world in recent decades. We can better understand a future debate if we understand more precisely the social location of the Promethean fatalist discourse in the religious world.

The choice of which discourse to use when discussing an RGT is determined by whether the new situation of an RGT is considered to be the same as a situation for which a discourse has been used for previously. To take an obvious example, some respondents use discourses from previous discussions of abortion to discuss abortion with the interviewer. Promethean fatalism does not just enter a respondent's mind with our conversation, but was rather used previously ("use" would include the more specific phenomena of being "taught" a discourse). It is a discourse that some religious traditions use repeatedly, for myriad situations, and that some religious traditions essentially never use. People who are embedded in particular traditions will then have more or less experience with using a discourse, making it more likely that they will use it. The survey shows that, although the Promethean discourse is more likely used by any participating Christian than by those who do not participate in religion, it is most likely to be used by the conservative Protestants and the traditionalist Catholics than by members of the other traditions in this study.[44]

This is consistent with what we know from scholarly generalizations about previous discourse use in these traditions. These generalizations are, to use my language, descriptions of the repeated use of a particular discourse for situations that their members encounter. For example, Mennonites would encounter an immanent war and see this situation as the same as previous instances where their pacifist discourse was used. Scholars would say that Mennonites are in a pacifist religious tradition. Catholics would encounter an immanent war and conclude that the war is just, because it had particular features. Scholars would then call Catholicism a just war Christian tradition. I cannot show the origins of discourse use in a tradition, which may have been hundreds or even thousands of years ago, but I can show that the discourse use I identify in this and other chapters is consistent with previous use in the tradition.

Because of the theological content of the Promethean fatalism discourse, it is obvious that the religious would use Promethean fatalism more than the nonreligious. The more interesting question is why conservative Protestants and traditionalist Catholics would be more likely than more liberal Christians to use this discourse. We can gain leverage on this question by reviewing a classic distinction within Christianity, which is between immanent and transcendent notions of God. In an immanent notion of God, God is present in the world, interacting with humans. In a transcendent view, God is radically other, and thus beyond human relationships or understanding. Both of these tendencies exist within each Christian tradition, but some traditions emphasize one view over the other.

Catholics have been classically considered to hold a more immanent notion of God. For example, the Catholic Church teaches transubstantiation and the interventions of the saints.[45] Protestants are classically thought to hold a transcendent notion of God, believing, for example, that God is not physically present during the Eucharist.[46] To extrapolate to the case of RGTs, an immanent God would be involved and interested in the details of your genetic make-up. A transcendent God is not concerned with such details. An immanent God could be threatened by your stealing technologies; a transcendent God could never be threatened by a human.

Catholics adhere to the belief in an immanent God. For example, consider this missive about Fathers' Day from the Catholic weekly *Our Daily Visitor*. The author asks, "What does it mean to call God 'Father'?"

The "the supreme Being is not just "King of the Universe" or "Master" but "Father," [and] he desires that we have a close, familiar relationship with Him.

We expect a dad to have an intimate, affectionate relationship with his children, to spend "quality time" with them. To call God "Father" means, then, that he is near to us, intimately concerned with us, fond of us, even crazy about us. He is not the distant, clockmaker God of Thomas Jefferson and the Deists. No, the God whom Jesus calls Father cares about us and knows us intimately. "Every hair on your head is numbered (Mat 10:30)." He loves us more than we love ourselves and knows us better than we know ourselves.[47]

Although Protestants have traditionally been considered as having a transcendent focus, in recent decades, conservative Protestants have moved toward more immanent beliefs. A study of evangelical popular texts found that "the traditional transcendent imagery concerning God has been minimized in favor of emphasis on depictions of some of God's immanent features: his benevolence, love and sympathy for humankind. Easily accessible, God is patiently concerned with the extraordinary and daily problems of people. He is tolerant of human foibles and errors, and democratic in his treatment of mortal beings."[48] This concept reaches its peak in Pentecostalism, where God heals the illnesses of people one by one. It is easy to see how people who regularly use the discourse of an immanent God would use this discourse for discussing RGTs and say that God had planned their children's genetic composition and decides who is to have which genetic trait.

This degree of a belief in immanence is not found in the mainline Protestant tradition. It is probably not a strict belief in immanence or transcendence that is at issue here, but rather a lack of belief that God intervenes actively in the world. Mainline Protestants are, after all, the ones who have traditionally minimized the supernatural aspects of the Christian narrative where God or Jesus intervened in nature. This debate is also foreign to the Jews whom we interviewed. Although God was immanent in the events described in the Torah, our Jewish interviewees do not have an orientation where God currently intervenes in human affairs. I would describe them as believing that God, through God's representatives, established the Jewish tradition, which is to be followed.

Conclusion

This chapter has partially answered the questions I posed in the introduction concerning why religious people were more opposed to RGTs and whether an RGT debate would be ineffective because people would not actually deliberate due to a lack of shared discourses. First, I have described the discourses of opposition to RGTs that involve God, nature, and humans. Philosophers, social scientists, and bioethicists generally want to avoid the naturalistic fallacy, where nature is looked to as a source of ethics. In contrast, most of the people with whom we spoke invoked nature at some point to justify an ethical stance toward RGTs. Of course, there are many different discourses of nature. I first examined a secular discourse about "nature," where the natural approach was the safest; thus, "nature" should be deferred to unless there was a compelling reason. Another discourse about the relationship among nature, humans, and God is the hubris discourse, where there is no technology that is inherently to be left to God. These discourses were primarily used by the (relative) proponents to oppose enhancements. Another discourse, natural law, used by some of the Catholic strong opponents of RGTs, holds that there is a way that nature should be—not necessarily the same as it is—that we should follow. An example would be that humans should be free of disease.

Other academic writings, as well as the writings of participants in elite debates about RGTs, often imply a Promethean fatalist discourse. That is, God has some talent that humans can, but should not, steal, as well as a plan for each person that should not be modified. While this is not the most commonly used discourse it is the discourse that is used by those who are the most opposed to RGTs.

How Promethean fatalism is used stands in contrast to how many academics and activists say it is used. Academic proponents of RGTs like John Harris assume that religious opposition to RGTs is driven by a hyper-Promethean fatalism, where God has assigned no powers to humans. In domain language, Harris presumes an issue domain called "everything that God created," where religious people will use the Promethean fatalist discourse. But, in actuality, those ordinary religious citizens who use the Promethean fatalist discourse consider healing disease to be part of the human agenda and not a task reserved for God, even though God created or allowed disease. For most people, human genetic engineering for cystic fibrosis was not a case where we should "trust God," but rather a case where we humans should act. For others, every RGT, except RGTs for enhancement, were similar to human genetic engineering for cystic fibrosis. In other words, the issue domain where Promethean fatalism is used is not "all that God created," but rather "all that God created excluding health promotion or medicine." This is the meaning of the Promethean fatalism discourse.

How the respondents talk during the interviews has implications for future deliberations about RGTs. First, it does appear that the pro-lifers use the Promethean fatalism discourse to discuss not only abortion and RGTs that destroy embryos but also RGTs that do not implicate embryos, such as sperm sorting and human genetic engineering. This suggests that there is an issue domain that I call "opposition to genetic control" that includes abortion for cystic fibrosis and these RGTs—abortion and RGTs would be "the same." Scholarly predictions of a merger of the abortion and RGT issues for the pro-lifers seem to be correct.

However, I also show that the concern that this merger will result in a lack of shared discourse is overstated. While some on the non–pro-life side are indeed using different discourses, like the hubris discourse, others are using the same Promethean fatalist discourse as the pro-life opponents. The interviews show that the smaller group of non–pro-lifers use the Promethean fatalist discourse to oppose abortion and the same RGTs as the pro-lifers. This suggests an extremely porous discursive wall between the sides of the abortion debate. The larger group of non–pro-lifers use the Promethean fatalist discourse to oppose enhancements. This shared discourse across the supposed divide would be the basis on which to build a discussion about related issues, such as pre-implantation genetic diagnosis for health reasons where the two sides disagree.

CHAPTER FIVE

Human Dignity and Equality of Treatment

The whole philosophy of Hell rests on recognition of the axiom that one thing is not another thing, and, especially, that one self is not another self. My good is my good, and your good is your good. What one gains another loses.—C. S. Lewis[1]

The term human dignity has been used extensively in bioethical debates about reproductive genetic technologies (RGTs), but not always clearly.[2] For secular bioethics the religious origin of the term has been refracted through Kant to come to mean respecting the autonomy of people to make their own decisions.[3] Therefore, secular bioethics in the United States studiously avoids the term human dignity but embraces the more specific term of "autonomy." However, conservatives, who are typically the opponents of RGTs, continue to use the term "dignity."

This term has become a marker of conservative bioethics in contrast with liberal bioethics. In fact, dignity is so central to evangelical bioethics that the term is in the names of their research centers, such as the Center for Bioethics and Human Dignity. Similarly, unlike any of its predecessors, the bioethics commission of the George W. Bush administration—which had more conservative commissioners than previous commissions—extensively used the language of dignity. For example, their published reports included *Human Cloning and Human Dignity: An Ethical Inquiry* and *Human Dignity and Bioethics.*[4]

In this chapter, I show that the religious public opposes RGTs using a number of discourses about "dignity," but there is a particular version of this discourse that is used by the stronger opponents of RGTs. As in the previous chapter, I separately examine those who do and do not use the embryonic life discourse to evaluate whether those who are on the pro-life side of the abortion debate have a broader issue domain that includes abortion and RGTs, and whether there are shared discourses across the divide of the abortion debate.

Human Dignity and Conservative Bioethics

The academic debates about dignity can help us understand the meaning of what the respondents are saying. Among religious bioethicists, one of the primary sources of the idea of human dignity is the Jewish and Christian traditions that attribute a supreme worth to humanity because humans have a special relationship with God: they are *Imago Dei*, made in God's image.[5] Since we are all made in God's image, we have equal value; therefore, we should be treated equally. According to one summary: "it is this conception that is in view, for example, when we refer to the inviolability of human dignity, to the intrinsic moral worth of humanity, or when we speak of inalienable human rights founded upon and expressive of that dignity."[6]

Of course, this notion of dignity does not produce explicit instructions for the ethics of RGTs, with Christians disagreeing about what dignity means and which humans are to be treated equally.[7] It also does not define what a human is, which is central when discussing issues involving embryos, where the humanity of an embryo is a central issue. However, if one accepts that embryos are persons, then they are deserving of equal dignity in this tradition. Dignity then means, at a minimum, that they are treated like all other humans and not destroyed.

Many of the academic and activist opponents of RGTs say that the reason conservatives are opposed (or should be opposed) to RGTs is that they believe in human dignity. For example, conservative bioethicist Eric Cohen claims that conservatives are opposed to RGTs because they are defenders of "the dignity of the weak":

> But conservatives also defend the dignity of those who will never run or swim or compose or fight, and the dignity of those embryos that cannot yet do these things. And we argue against those who claim that the very lack of these powers makes such lives not worth living or protecting and against those who are

tempted to seek equality by aborting (or euthanizing) the imperfects. . . . We are
for unconditional love and conditional excellence.[8]

Similarly, theologian Gilbert Meilaender's conclusion about RGTs where
we are "designing our descendants" is that "not only is the meaning of
childhood distorted but the meaning of parenthood as well. Selective
abortion means selective acceptance. The unconditional character of ma-
ternal and paternal love is replaced by choice, quality control, and an only
conditional acceptance."[9] His conclusion is premised on love, which also
means treating other humans as having unconditional value:

> There remains love, the greatest of the virtues. Love signifies approval, and . . .
> our own love mirrors the creative love of God, which bestows on us the divine
> word of approval. Love therefore is . . . a way of turning to another and saying,
> "It's good that you exist; it's good that you are in this world." As we hope to be-
> come people who can love our own children in this way, so we would want them,
> in turn, to be people who can love as they have been loved-with an affirmation
> that is not conditioned upon the qualities of the loved one.

While not mentioned by Cohen or Meilaender, their invocation of human dignity and treating all humans as equals actually focuses on a particular version of dignity and equality. I find two major discourses of dignity
and equal treatment used by the religious public when opposing RGTs,
distinguished by how broad their social vision is when determining who
is to be treated equally. Does equal treatment mean equal treatment between any two hypothetical people? This is the discourse used by religious
and conservative bioethicists, as well as by the respondents who are the
stronger opponents of RGTs. Or, does it mean equal treatment between
groups in society, such as races or classes? This is used by the (relative)
proponents to oppose enhancements.[10] The former I will call the discourse
of individual dignity/equality, and the latter social dignity/equality.

Social Dignity/Equality

Consider our conversation with Martin, a liberal Catholic, who is in favor
of almost all the applications and technologies. We first discuss whether
a couple should use preimplantation genetic diagnosis for cystic fibrosis,
which is where a number of embryos are created and those with cystic

fibrosis are discarded, and those free of cystic fibrosis are implanted in the woman. To this he says, "Absolutely! Why wouldn't they? . . . It's better to ensure that you will not bring a child with cystic fibrosis into the world for all that suffering and possible death. If you can ensure that through science, why wouldn't you? Absolutely!"

He supports every technology and application until we reach preimplantation genetic diagnosis for intelligence, which is the first technology of which he is not an enthusiastic supporter:

> Um . . . [*pause*] . . . well we are sort of now touching on the Dr. Mengele master race of . . . of higher IQ. But there's a wonderful movie called *Gattaca*, which addresses this issue of the super gene pool. I guess down the road people in the future people may be doing this. It seems to be an adjunct and an outgrowth of all the more efficacious ways of using science to improve the quality of life. I suppose that there will always be people that are trying to create the quote unquote master race. There's a woman selling her eggs, a woman with an IQ of 180, [for] $50,000 an egg. You know, this stuff is going to go on in the brave new world. There's little that we can do about it. I don't know if it's wrong or we should outlaw it. . . . It seems to me frivolous. . . . Are you only going to love your child who's got a 160 IQ?

People using this discourse often invoke the Nazis and their idea of the master race of blue-eyed, tall, beautiful people as the previous situation that fits with RGTs. (Interestingly, they also do not tend to note that the Nazis would have wanted to eliminate people with genetic diseases.) Many of the respondents also had concerns similar to those expressed in the 1997 movie *Gattaca*, which Martin had obviously seen. In the dystopian society portrayed in this movie, the people are genetically screened to determine their life chances, and society discriminates against them accordingly. The main character in the movie dreams of being a professional space traveler, but the society is structured so that people with his genetic make-up are appointed to mundane tasks.

Martin then says he prefers "the natural approach. I don't ever intend to get a nose job or a . . . you know an eye tuck or whatever. I prefer to go natural. Same with childbirth. I think it's better when possible to let nature take its course . . . if it's not to improve the safety of the child." He is, as we might expect, in favor of the health applications of human genetic engineering, where embryos are modified to remove or add genes, changing the genetic make-up of future generations. "Should the couple do this?"

we asked. "Absolutely! Why would somebody even ask?" he responded. But, as with preimplantation genetic diagnosis, he was also leery of using human genetic engineering to improve children's intelligence.

Chad, also drew the line at using RGTs to improve intelligence. He had no particular concerns about destroying embryos and was in favor of most of the technologies. For example, he sees preimplantation genetic diagnosis as akin to the natural variability that occurs in getting pregnant "the old-fashioned way," saying, "If they're interested in being parents to begin with and just by natural selection, there is a chance of literally thousands of different types of babies being born from the same couple and nonetheless ultimately one is born. So there is virtually no difference in this process. It eliminates the problem of cystic fibrosis before it ever is an issue."

He felt similarly about all the applications, until we discussed using preimplantation genetic diagnosis for intelligence. To that scenario he responded:

> It's a different issue because now the issue has changed because now it has gone from an issue of eliminating hardships, handicaps, diseases, to enhancement and of course, that was one of the problems we had with Mr. Hitler. So would that be a process that would be available to everyone and if it were, would that be the best solution available? Good question. I guess probably most people would be very tempted to use that and so I would guess I'm probably, if put in that position, would probably choose to do that as well.

Chad is weighing his concern with creating social groups by their intelligence and treating them differently, although he concludes in the end that he would probably use this RGT to do the same.

Clare, one of the secular people with whom we spoke, was in favor of most of the technologies and applications, yet expresses her worries about an application—even though she ultimately approves of it—by using the secular nature discourse. With preimplantation genetic diagnosis for cystic fibrosis, she says:

> It doesn't sound much fun, but yeah, I think that that's fine. It's an opportunity to, you know, . . . at least it's giving the child a chance. Just because it's an abnormal way of doing it, I don't see any problem with that. . . . I mean it's not the natural way. So, you want things to be natural when you do something like that. . . . I don't have any strong feelings, you know, like moral feelings against

it because if these people are in that kind of situation, then they should deserve to have whatever options they could get to—to help them have a baby that's healthy.

She draws her line at preimplantation genetic diagnosis for obesity, concluding that "obesity doesn't seem like it's that debilitating of a disease when you talk about some of these other things that we're talking about. So maybe it doesn't warrant [the use of preimplantation genetic diagnosis]. I mean earlier there was that feeling that I had that this isn't natural."

In addition to her secular nature discourse, Clare uses the social dignity/equality discourse, saying that the technologies will not be available to everyone in society:

> Well, first of all, who's going to be able to do this? It's going to be people that have money, probably. I doubt that insurance companies are going to cover this kind of stuff. So when you really think about a race of superhumans, it's not going to be a race of superhumans, it's going to be a race of rich superhumans. Then there's going to be the people that don't have the money to do that kind of stuff. They're, you know, going to be disadvantaged because if you think, "Now I can . . . put 50 IQ points on this kid and this kid's going to be stronger and faster and all this kind of stuff," well look what you've done to society by doing that.

RGTs could create social classes of superintelligent persons, which would restructure society. Those who use this discourse hear of RGTs and draw an analogy to previous situations where they have used this discourse—most commonly in situations of class or race inequality. Clearly, for example, Clare has class inequality in mind in her narrative of the haves and the have nots. They then use the same discourse for the new situation of RGTs that they use for these earlier situations.

Individual Dignity/Equality

The individual dignity/equality discourse is associated with greater opposition to RGTs.[11] This discourse claims that it is wrong to pick and choose between any two particular people because of a characteristic, because we should all be equal. The problem is then to examine two particular people (or embryos) and pick between them. The analogy here would be similar to picking a particular job applicant because he or she is white, and not to a society that systematically discriminates in favor of whites. Because the individual dignity/equality discourse is used by the strongest opponents of RGTs, I separately examine the pro-lifers and the non–pro-lifers to evaluate the concerns about the effectiveness of a future RGT debate.

Individual Dignity/Equality among the Pro-lifers

In table 3 in chapter 3, 90 percent of the pro-life, stronger opponents of RGTs also use the individual dignity/equality discourse for RGTs in general, although we cannot tell from the survey for which or for how many RGTs they would use this discourse. During the in-depth interviews, these people often start with intertwining the embryonic life and individual dignity/equality discourses when discussing technologies that potentially harm embryos, and then, as the interview progressed, shift to only the latter discourse to discuss RGTs that do not harm embryos.

For example, Jane is a nontraditional evangelical who is definitely opposed to destroying embryos or fetuses and clearly states that life begins at conception. She initially says she would never have an abortion, so amniocentesis is unacceptable, but she does not say why. When we discuss preimplantation genetic diagnosis, her initial objections become clear when she talks about what happens to the embryos not selected for implantation: "Yeah. Is it just like flushed, or? It's still, there's still life. I think there is."

She could logically continue with the embryonic life discourse to discuss all the preimplantation genetic diagnosis scenarios, but instead she uses the individual inequality discourse:

> I really don't have a problem with in vitro. But [I do with] the pick-and-choose factor [involved with preimplantation genetic diagnosis], because that's what makes so many of us different. We're all different and who is to say that maybe this child when he or she is eighteen or twenty-two years old comes up and does some major, something, or is very intelligent before they hit that thirty-year mark, or saves someone's life in a house fire?

Later, she continued:

> Well, just because maybe this person or this child has that sort of a problem, who is to say I don't like this hair color. Where is the limit as to what you say you can or you cannot do? I don't know if you can determine hair color,

and all like that, but who is to say at one point you're going to . . . What is the cutoff?

She does not want to treat people—or potential people, depending on your view—unequally by letting some live and some die. When asked about preimplantation genetic diagnosis for Alzheimer's, she skips the embryonic life discourse again and says, "If it's not right in one case for one sort of a disease, who is to say what disease is worse than the other?" All are to be treated equally. When asked if one of these applications of preimplantation genetic diagnosis is worse than another, she says she sees no difference "because you're picking and choosing still. It's like going to the grocery store saying I don't want this or I want this. A can of beans is a can of beans." This is the imagery used by those who use this discourse—they do not speak of the stratified societies like those who use the social dignity/equality discourse, but of having to pick between people like products on a shelf.

A can of beans is a can of beans is a nice everyday metaphor for saying that all humans are the same to Jane; thus, to treat them differently by choosing between them is wrong. She disapproves of preimplantation genetic diagnosis for sex selection "because the male embryos are gone" and initially approves of sperm sorting for sex "because they're not terminating a life." However, in Jane's decision about which previous situation sperm sorting is analogous, she notes that she sees a "conflict" with what she has said: "Because here, now, they're saying that they want a female and why is it okay for them to have a female, when it's not okay for them to have this one with a disease? But, they've already had two children that are male. It's somewhat of a problem, obviously." Sperm sorting does not fit the previous situations where she uses the embryonic life discourse, and she cannot decide whether picking sperm by sex is the same situation as picking for disease, which she has previously used the individual dignity/equality discourse to oppose.

When we turn to human genetic engineering for cystic fibrosis, she is clearly checking to see if her embryonic life discourse fits when she says it would be "very tempting. If I knew I was not harming any other life and could make this one healthy and my future generations . . . I'd probably consider it. I'd look into it. I'd want to research it. Yes." As with the Promethean fatalist discourse, the individual dignity/equality discourse does not fit with what these respondents perceive to be the salient features of human genetic engineering for cystic fibrosis. Even though human genetic engineering for cystic fibrosis would produce the same outcome as preimplantation genetic diagnosis for cystic fibrosis—essentially picking and choosing the type of child you will have—this is not seen as analogous to other situations of picking and choosing.

As we move to discussing human genetic engineering for other traits, with the embryonic life discourse no longer in her consideration because the lives of embryos are not at stake, she worries that the technology would be applied beyond diseases and reinvokes the individual equality discourse, saying, "Just because I said it would be tempting doesn't necessarily mean that it's right. Again, where are the limits going to be? What's going to stop? . . . We're going to prevent this disease. But, maybe there's something else. Well, let's have it so the future children will be sterile so there's no more children? Let's cut down the population. Who's to say that something like that couldn't happen?" Once we are no longer discussing disease, she is back to using the same individual dignity/equality discourse she uses for abortion, suggesting that they are in the same domain and thus largely the same.

Kathleen, a mainline Protestant teacher, is similar and says, "I don't believe in abortion." When discussing preimplantation genetic diagnosis for cystic fibrosis, she states that

> I think pretty much babies are miracles and they are God-given and you would do everything in your power to make, you know, your child healthy by watching—you know, no smoking, no drinking, whatever. But I do think some of our families that have special children, it turns they are even more special than special . . . And most [families] would not trade them for anything. We had several in the church and they are very special children and as long as you get the support you need. But I don't know that I would pick and choose [*laugh*]. You know, this egg and sperm is going to go down the drain and this one is not.

She is making an analogy between selectively destroying embryos and a previous experience with the "special children" in her church that their families would not trade for anything. Indeed, earlier she mentioned that a baby in her church had died of cystic fibrosis, and the baby "meant a lot to [the parents] just for the ten or eleven months they had her. She meant a lot to the church." The salient feature of this new situation of preimplantation genetic diagnosis with which she has been presented seems to be that, like abortion, you could destroy valuable people like the child in her church who had cystic fibrosis, when we all should have equal value.

When the conversation turned to preimplantation genetic diagnosis for early onset Alzheimer's disease, she says:

> I don't think I would recommend that. I think people playing God pretty much to do that. Now if the baby was already in development and they tested it or it helped with their medical treatment or early diagnoses or whatever, but to actually choose a child: not this egg or not this egg or not this egg for different reasons, I just—I would have a real hard time with that.

After stating her opposition to other applications of preimplantation genetic diagnosis, she says that "there are no circumstances that I would choose five Petri dishes with [*laugh*] eggs and sperm and pick and choose which one you wanted. There's no way that I would do that."

Like many strong opponents of RGTs, Kathleen switches among the Promethean fatalism, individual dignity/equality, and meaningful suffering discourses. With preimplantation genetic diagnosis for sex selection, she uses a bit of the Promethean fatalist discourse by saying, "No. I think you get what you get. . . . [you can't] just say 'we want a girl'." With sperm sorting for sex, she continues with Promethean fatalism:

> It's tampering. It's tampering with nature. . . . I think you can tamper by doing the best that you can, you know, eating the best you can, being as healthy as you can, whatever, that kind of tampering. But controlling everything, to me, is something that a lot of it—you know, God does it. We just don't have that. I don't think we should have that power to tamper with what's been forever.

The discussion turned to human genetic engineering for cystic fibrosis, which in my depiction does not result in the destruction of embryos. Prior to the discussions with ordinary religious people, I would have thought that this situation would be analogous to previous situations where individuals were treated unequally because a type of person is not being allowed to exist in future generations. In my opinion, you are picking and choosing. But, like other respondents, she does not see human genetic engineering for cystic fibrosis as an analogous situation to abortion for cystic fibrosis and does not use the same discourse. Like others, she appears to put it in a "medicine" domain.

She is, however, more equivocal than others. She says that human genetic engineering for cystic fibrosis "on the one hand, sounds really good." She says, "I think [the technology] will be here and a lot of people will want it for those serious diseases, you know, to be eradicated like polio was eradicated which of course is not genetic. . . . But to eradicate a disease like that, I think a lot of people will think that's wonderful." Unlike others, she is still weighing the analogy she is making between medical care and treating people unequally due to some personal characteristic. She then sighs and says, "I just don't see choosing this baby over this baby kind of thing but I do think it will come to that point where they will eradicate it." By the time we move to the next question, which concerns human genetic engineering for obesity, she is firm in her one-word answer, "No," which she continues for all other applications of human genetic engineering that she considers not for diseases, with the analogy to a previous situation of inequality clearly in place. In regards to cloning, she returns to the Promethean fatalist discourse, concluding that "I just don't like any of the tampering with nature and what's a God-given miracle of having children. I just don't agree with the tampering."

Individual Dignity/Equality among the Non–pro-lifers

The individual dignity/equality discourse is also used by the non–pro-lifers—those who do not use the embryonic life discourse. Again, there are those who reach the same conclusions as those on the other side of the supposed discursive divide—and use all but the embryonic life discourse do to so—suggesting a very porous divide. There are also the (relative) proponents who only agree with the strong opponents about enhancements, but do use the individual dignity/equality discourse to do so, suggesting a moderately porous divide. For example Meghan, a retired Catholic woman who attends mass weekly, clearly does not use the embryonic life discourse. She was not categorically opposed to technologies that destroyed embryos and was in favor of using preimplantation genetic diagnosis for cystic fibrosis. Of course, almost no one with whom we spoke thought abortion was without moral consequence. Like others, she clearly is not enthusiastic about abortion, and when asked about using abortion with amniocentesis, she said:

And of course, no one knows how [the couple] will react to a challenge or something in their life that's unexpected. Some people rise to the occasion; some people don't. I guess it would have to be an extreme case of one of those things I described before I would think it would be better for them to abort because they simply would not be able to deal with the child like that. . . .

I would be reluctant because I don't think I believe that a fetus is a human being at the moment of conception but by fifteen weeks I think you do have . . . I mean who am I to say when the soul enters the body, I don't know, but here I think you have . . . that would be roughly three months, a three-month fetus so at a sense you're at the end of the first trimester.

Like many other Americans, she has a developmental view of fetal personhood—an embryo is not a person, but a three-month-old fetus is. She approves of preimplantation genetic diagnosis for cystic fibrosis and says, "Well again, I guess I just don't feel that at eight cells, you have a human being where if you have someone two or three months along then I think there is new life present and that's probably why I wouldn't."

She approves of applications of preimplantation genetic diagnosis that are designed to alleviate the most severe health problems, but she stops at using this technology for obesity, saying, "I don't think it goes with Christian teaching. I guess what I'm saying is Christ didn't pick perfect people, he didn't pick people who were necessarily smart or rich or had certain genes, and we don't know what genes they had and that . . . and I suppose the supposition behind all of this . . . I don't know is it that a person who is not obese or a person who does not develop . . . is somehow more valuable." This opposition to picking and choosing is the hallmark of using the individual dignity/equality discourse and is used not only by those who also use the embryonic life discourse but also by people like Meghan, who do not.

She explicitly connects to what she sees as one of the core messages in the Christian tradition, that Christ was and is there for everybody, and not just, as she puts it, "the perfect people." Everyone has value, and these technologies violate this idea. Of course, participants in the scholarly bioethics debate like Cohen or Meilaender would point out that people with cystic fibrosis have equal value, but this is not how the (relative) proponents see it.

She later approves of human genetic engineering for cystic fibrosis. While it could be argued that this is picking the type of person to bring into existence as well, she does not see it as matching her discourse of dignity/equality, but rather avoiding disease seems paramount. When we asked if she had "any concerns about the technology of being able to remove the cystic fibrosis from the family tree forever?" she responded, "I don't think I do because it's an illness. The limitation on the life of the human being that's going to be born. It isn't like brown hair or blue eyes." She reiterated that she was opposed to human genetic engineering for obesity or intelligence, for the same individual equality reasons she gave earlier.

Phil is opposed to abortion for cystic fibrosis without referencing the embryonic life discourse, and he is one with a more porous boundary with those on the other side of the communicative divide. Abortion for cystic fibrosis is wrong because it is a situation of treating individuals unequally. If the couple were pregnant, says Phil, instead of conducting amniocentesis, "They should, I mean, go for it and love the child as if it didn't have cystic fibrosis. I mean, all you can do is love your kids as much as you can and do the best for them and if they're already pregnant, I don't think—I think abortion is wrong."

When asked about preimplantation genetic diagnosis for cystic fibrosis, Phil appears to be one of the many respondents with a developmental notion of fetal personhood, and does not use the embryonic life discourse, because he does not seem to be concerned with the inevitable death of embryos that occurs with preimplantation genetic diagnosis. Rather, he agonizes over whether to apply a discourse about health or individual dignity/equality. He replies:

> I don't know. I don't know. I don't know [*laugh*]. That's definitely an ethical question. Should you pick a designer baby? On one hand, it's certainly more convenient for the parents—you know, no parents ever imagined their child growing up with difficulties and having disease and what not. But on the other hand, I question the ethics of being able to choose your kid. . . . But on the other hand, it would certainly . . . I mean, given the medical expenses and what not and the pain, I don't know.

Note that the lives of embryos are not part of his decision-making process. When we asked, "What's the most problematic for you about this method?" He replied with the following:

> Being able to choose is the most problematic. I mean, how do you say you're going to love one child less than the other? You know, I love this child that doesn't have cystic fibrosis more and it's going to be happier than having the child who does have it. How does one argue that? I don't know. I don't see how you can. A normal child's life will be easier and longer but on the other hand, you may be missing out on a really special soul.

He makes an analogy to a very personal previous situation when selecting his individual dignity/equality discourse, saying:

It would horrify me to know that my parents said, "Oh well, you know, we didn't want you. We were hoping for a designer baby." Or "you have a back problem. We wished we would have done something about it to fix it." There is always that "what if" if you don't . . . My mother had a miscarriage after [an event] and because she had that miscarriage, she was able to have my [sibling] afterwards. So I just can't imagine not having my [sibling] around. That this special person whom I love, what would this other person be like? Would I have the same relationship? I don't know.[12]

He is opposed to other uses of preimplantation genetic diagnosis. As for using preimplantation genetic diagnosis to select the sex of a child, he says "Absolutely not," that this is like having "designer children. You're not going shopping at a store [*laugh*]. It's not like you go 'well no, I don't like this blouse. It's pink and it's going to shrink so I'm going to go with this other one.' You're having a kid! Like again, you're passing up an opportunity for nature to take its course." He continues:

We're given this ability to create and that's a wonderful thing. I think that we would in a sense be abusing that creation by deciding, "I don't want this child. This child's going to have a disease." Or "I want a boy. I want a girl." I mean, that's just ridiculous. Where does it stop? When are we going to say, "Well this boy is only going to be 5'5", I want my son to be at least 5'10". That's ridiculous, you know? "My son would live happier if he was 5'10". I mean, that's asinine. I just can't believe that people would put so little value on human life as to decide on making changes in the way that, you know, we live our lives now.

He carries through with his individual dignity/equality discourse when discussing sperm sorting to select for sex, which does not involve embryos. He says that sperm sorting is better than using preimplantation genetic diagnosis to determine sex because it is "more naturalistic . . . But still, they are still sorting out male and female and again, I still think that goes with the designer baby. . . . I still would have ethical problems with that. It's still choosing your baby."

Although he was torn about preimplantation genetic diagnosis for cystic fibrosis, he is more enthusiastic about human genetic engineering for cystic fibrosis, invoking an analogy to previous discussions of medicine. He says that this technology "goes along the same lines as medical technology now. There are things that we can do now that we couldn't do when I was growing up or when we were growing up. You know, the child is ready to survive or we've given it a certain operation or whatever is so much greater in certain circumstances and that would certainly go along the same lines. You know, if we can make things better, why not?"

Human genetic engineering for obesity is different, because unlike cystic fibrosis obesity is "not a life-threatening disease." Creating a flower metaphor to articulate his concern with picking and choosing, he says:

> Obesity, while some view as a disease, I think it's just a different type of flower and regarding of life. I mean, then maybe one could argue "well maybe cystic fibrosis is, too." But I don't know if it's better to have a bunch of flowers and a bunch that die than to have less flowers, less a variety of flowers but flowers that live a lot longer. It's kind of what would you pick? Would you pick the flower, the plant, that's going to live through the winter or are you going to pick the one that dies and you'll have to replant next spring?

His hesitation with human genetic engineering for intelligence "is that again you devalue the ones that are not able to have that procedure done or have been born and are not smart."

Finally, consider our conversation with Andrew. He is a salesman and a traditional evangelical. In our conversation about whether a couple should try to have children if they know they are carriers for cystic fibrosis, Andrew starts with the individual dignity/equality discourse. He says that they should just have a child because:

> I'm not sure that life is measured in length as much as it's measured in breadth. I have a good friend whose [relative] was born not able to speak; not able to move and pretty much what some people would call a vegetable . . . and yeah when you realize the impact that his [relative][13] had on his family, it was really significant and it was a worthwhile life, while we may not necessarily call it . . . society may not measure it exactly that way.

Like many others, he is also weighing the issue of disease. Andrew follows his statement about the equality of people by talking about the odds that the parents would pass on cystic fibrosis, saying:

> So the other thing is that when you look at it, one in four, I mean if it was 100 percent then maybe you'd say gosh do I want to raise a child with those kind of handicaps and what will that mean to my life, on the other hand you may have

a child or two that doesn't have that problem. Should they have four children, I don't know. I'd go with the roll of the dice.

If it were 100 percent that the child would have cystic fibrosis, then perhaps intervention would be justified.

For amniocentesis, Andrew returns to the equality discourse and says, "Yeah, I would go back to my initial statement to say that life is more than just a measured time span and that I think that all life, even severely handicapped life, is worthwhile and so that would be at least one answer." When it comes to preimplantation genetic diagnosis, he approves, apparently because it would have perfect certitude in avoiding a child with the disease. He quickly adds a comment that foreshadows the reemergence of the individual dignity/equality discourse for uses of preimplantation genetic diagnosis that he considers to not be about disease. He is concerned that the technology

> would be used in ways that weren't necessarily beneficial for society in terms of predetermining the sex of the baby, and predetermining the other characteristics of a child. If you hated blue eyes, well let's lose the ones with blue eyes. We can look at society's like China where so many young girls are given up for adoption because they want boys and realize that that may be a sociological preference that ultimately I'm not sure it's that it's really the society's choice to make.

He states his opposition to RGTs most clearly when it comes to intelligence. While his concern with avoiding disease in the case of cystic fibrosis outweighs his discourse of individual dignity/equality with enhancements like intelligence, the discourse of individual dignity/equality reemerges:

> I guess I would probably say that each child is a gift from God and that while no two children are the same, that each being the gifts that they are would bring their abilities and their skills and their intelligence levels to help and better society and that's it's not always necessarily just a matter of intelligence quotients but it may be compassion and caring and things that are actually a good measure of that. . . . In the context of a Christian faith [it is important] to be able to give another measure besides intelligence to measure on.

With sperm sorting for sex determination, Andrew continues with the individual dignity/equality discourse by saying, "It's almost the same as deciding which egg you're going to implant based on sex so I guess I would want to opt not to do that." As we discuss human genetic engineering for cystic fibrosis, he reaches for analogies to medical experiences in his past to inform his choice of discourse. He says that the hypothetical couple should use the technology. He says, "I don't really have a concern with it. I mean whether you could fix it . . . when I look at my friend's kids who have cleft palettes, I know that I have friends who chose not to have another child because of that genetic predisposition. [They opted for] adoption there. If they could have fixed that in utero, they would have, absolutely! And if they could have fixed that about themselves, they would have had other children themselves. Sure I'd do it."

Human genetic engineering for cystic fibrosis is in the health promotion domain (see fig. 3, chap. 1), and the individual dignity/equality discourse no longer fits for Andrew. However, when the conversation next turns to human genetic engineering for obesity, he opposes that because he does not consider it to be a disease, and he returns to his previous criteria for conditions that are not diseases. He is opposed to all other types of human genetic engineering.

Almost everyone is opposed to what they perceive to be enhancements. Those with the more permissive line between health and enhancements (such as stopping at improving intelligence) use the social dignity/equality discourse. Those with the less permissive line (such as stopping at marginal diseases such as deafness), use the same individual dignity/equality discourse as do the strongest opponents of RGTs. In the survey, 88 percent of the non–pro-lifer (relative) proponents of RGTs do use the individual dignity/equality discourse to oppose at least some RGTs.[14] Clearly, people on both sides of the abortion debate use this discourse for RGTs, and the interviews show more clearly for which RGTs this is the case. This is further evidence against the idea of a strong discursive divide over RGTs along the two sides of the abortion debate, as well as evidence against a strong divide between opponents and (relative) proponents of RGTs.

The Social Location of the Dignity/Equality Discourses

People in certain religious traditions are more likely to use particular discourses because they are taught to use these discourses for other situations. The obvious example is that many Catholics are taught the embryonic life discourse. In other religious traditions, members will, over the course of their lifetimes, hear people using the individual dignity/equality discourse for myriad situations and will tend to use it themselves.

The survey shows that while the individual dignity/equality discourse is more likely to be held by Christians who attend church than by the non-religious, there are few differences in use between Christian traditions.[15] We can look at generalizations about the Christian tradition to see how Christians have previously used this discourse.

In the narrative that Christians tell about the founding of their religion, Christianity emerged from Judaism as a universalistic alternative to a particularistic ethnic religion. Judaism was for the ethnic Jews, but Christianity was to be ethnically universal and, depending on how you want to interpret the tradition, was to not make distinctions based on race, sex, or economic class. All were to be treated the same, including your enemies. In one of the central biblical texts justifying a separation from Judaism, Paul writes to the church at Galatia, "There is no longer Jew or Greek, there is no longer slave or free, there is no longer male and female; for all of you are one in Christ Jesus."[16]

This can, and has been, like most other Bible passages, interpreted in many ways. One interpretation could be that Christians are to ignore these social distinctions when it comes to membership in the new religion, which clearly is at least advocated in principle in Christianity. Other theological strands also contribute to linking dignity and the rejection of inequalities. Continuing the distinction with Judaism central to the development of Christianity as a separate religion, the apostle Mark depicts Jesus as saying, when asked which of the commandments is most important:

> The first is, "Hear, O Israel: the Lord our God, the Lord is one; you shall love the Lord your God with all your heart, and with all your soul, and with all your mind, and with all your strength." The second is this, "You shall love your neighbor as yourself." There is no other commandment greater than these. (Mark 12:28–31, New Revised Standard Version)

This notion is not unique to Christianity, but Christians consider the second commandment above to be one of the central themes of the religion. You should treat your neighbor—generally considered to be all other humans—like you would like to be treated. So, we can see how Christians would repeatedly use this discourse for varied situations and thus have this discourse available to them.

Historians have claimed that this discourse has, to use my terminology, been repeatedly applied by Christians when they encounter new situations. For example, Hugh Heclo claims that Christians used the discourse of individual dignity/equality when faced with the situation of how to design the political system of the United States. He writes:

> Throughout the Bible God calls to humans by their personal names, often bypassing their tribal or other identities. In the New Testament this is radically reaffirmed with the poetic but still extraordinary claim that the hairs on each person's head are "numbered"—known to God not just in their collective sum, but each bar-coded, so to speak. Humans have inherent dignity and worth as individual, personally distinct beings.
>
> The importance of this individuation is overlooked in a common political science claim, generally to the effect that democracy assumes "the essential dignity of man." For whatever portion of American democracy has been influenced by Christianity, this is not true. Pagan philosophers, Enlightenment monarchs, aristocrats, and elites of all sorts have often espoused the essential dignity of man. In America democracy assumes, as Christianity declares, the essential dignity of each person, one at a time.[17]

While the individual dignity/equality discourse is more likely to be used for RGTs by the active Christians rather than by the nonreligious, the social dignity/equality discourse is used equally by all survey respondents, secular and religious, except by conservative Protestants, who are less likely to use it.[18] Why are conservative Protestants less likely to use this discourse for new situations? The answer lies in the different orientations to society of the different religious groups.

Catholic and Protestant Orientations to Society

At one time, sociologist Andrew Greeley regularly administered a survey to his undergraduate students, asking them how often they phone or email their parents and siblings. He found that Catholics are more likely than Protestants to keep in touch in this way.[19] He took this as evidence of Catholic communalism, the idea that Catholics think of themselves as embedded in community, whereas Protestants think of themselves more as individuals. This is a very commonly articulated notion in social theory and popular culture more generally. For example, at the turn of the last century, Emile Durkheim tried to explain geographic variation in different suicide rates by looking at the dominant religious group in each area.[20] The Catholics were more integrated into the society than the Protestants and therefore were considered to be less likely to commit suicide.

Catholic communalism is a part not only of Catholic culture but also of church teachings—that is, it is used repeatedly in the tradition. From a study of 284 papal encyclicals written between 1740 and 1987, Michael Schuck claims that

> internal to all the popes' social recommendations and judgments is a communitarian understanding of the self and society. Whether rooted in territorial custom, cosmological nature, or affective sentiment, the self is invariably defined by the totality of its relations with other beings and, particular, with other selves. Hence, the encyclicals constantly protest liberalism's enlightenment-inspired notion of the self as a radically unencumbered, autonomous chooser of ends.[21]

This has traditionally resulted in a Catholic concern with social justice, which has been explicated in various encyclicals and in the everyday activity of the Catholic church.[22]

Greeley believes that this official orientation in the church is associated with a particularly Catholic religious sensibility or culture. He writes, "The Catholic tends to see society as a 'sacrament' of God," so "society is 'natural' and 'good'." The Protestant, Greeley claims, "tends to see human society as 'God-forsaken' and therefore un-natural and oppressive. The individual stands over against society and is not integrated into it."[23]

This leads to a number of predictions for Greeley about how these different imaginations lead to different views on a more concrete level. Of the ones pertinent to this chapter, Greeley would predict that Catholics are more likely than Protestants to value social relationships and to value equality over freedom. Greeley has generally found in his research that this Catholic/Protestant difference in social imagination remains in the contemporary world.[24]

If Greeley is right, Catholics should be prone to seeing individuals as embedded in groups, and that entire groups can then be justly or unjustly treated. This would then make the social dignity/equality discourse used more often by Catholics and thus more available when these Catholics encounter a new situation like RGTs.

Other Protestants

Why would mainline Protestants have used the social dignity/equality discourse in the past and therefore be more likely to use it with RGTs? This discourse clearly has been repeatedly used among mainline Protestants. For example, the Social Gospel movement was a late nineteenth- and early-twentieth-century movement of mainline Protestants that focused on social problems, such as poverty, crime, child labor, and racial tensions. Proponents of the Social Gospel thought that people should not wait for the second coming of Christ, but should create the Kingdom of God on earth for the second coming to occur. This led to the idea that Christians should be deeply involved with solving the problems of society, which was associated with a more social view of the world. For example, one influential proponent, Walter Rauchenbush, argued that it is not only possible for individuals to sin but also for an entire social order to be sinful. It was not the individual in the slum who was sinful, but the social order that created the slum in the first place.[25] This is analogous to worries of picking between persons versus creating a *Gattaca*-like society.

While there are few people today who would explicitly claim allegiance to the Social Gospel movement, similar movements continue among mainline Protestants, making use of the social dignity/equality discourse. Whatever the source, it is reasonable to see that mainline Protestants have repeatedly used the social dignity/equality discourse.

The one remaining question is why conservative Protestants would less often use the social dignity/equality discourse. While the other religious traditions have a more communal orientation, the more individualistically oriented conservative Protestants view the world as an agglomeration of individuals, making it more difficult to see inequality between groups. Michael Emerson and Christian Smith found something similar when they report that evangelicals do not see systematic discrimination against blacks because their individualistic orientation to the world makes systematic thinking of inequality between groups impossible.[26]

Conclusion

The most socially expansive discourse about dignity and equality claims that we should treat entire groups equally, and RGTs threaten that social equality through creating genetically defined groups and creating yet another opportunity to treat those without money unequally. This discourse is more often used to oppose "enhancement" than "disease" applications of RGTs.

Many of the authors in the academic debates about RGTs portray a concern with what I call individual dignity/equality, that is, we should treat any two people equally, be they two people of different races, sexes, genetic conditions, or abilities. It is clear from talking with ordinary religious persons that the individual equality discourse is used by those who also use the embryonic life discourse more or less like it is used by these academics. People use the discourse to argue against treating embryos with cystic fibrosis differently than other embryos, and they also use the discourse for situations where embryos are not threatened, such as sperm sorting and human genetic engineering for enhancements. The analogy here is the other instances of opposition to picking and choosing between persons, and those who use this individual dignity/equality discourse are opposed to a broader range of RGTs and their applications. However, as with the other strongly oppositional discourses under close examination in this book, the individual dignity/equality discourse is not used to oppose human genetic engineering for cystic fibrosis.

This chapter reaches the same conclusion as the previous chapter concerning the conditions for an effective debate. First, it does appear that the pro-lifers use the individual dignity/equality discourse to discuss not only abortion and RGTs that threaten embryos but also RGTs that do not implicate embryos such as sperm sorting. In theory, this would make proponents of RGTs less likely to want to discuss RGTs with opponents, resulting in an ineffective debate, because the abortion and RGT issues would be seen as the same.

However, contrary to the expectation that there is no shared language with which to discuss RGTs with pro-lifers who have a merged abortion-RGT issue domain, in actuality the divide between pro-lifers and non–pro-lifers is porous. As with Promethean fatalism, the interviews show that the smaller group of non–pro-lifers, who reach the same conclusions about RGTs as those who *do* use the embryonic life discourse, also use the same discourses—except embryonic life—as those on the other side of the divide. This suggests a very porous divide and that deliberation is definitely possible. The larger group of non–pro-lifers do not use the individual dignity/equality discourse to oppose all RGTs, but only those that they consider to be enhancements. But, shared discourses on the same and closely related issues remain across the abortion divide. We now turn to the evaluation of the final oppositional discourse that emerged from the interviews.

CHAPTER SIX

Meaningful Suffering

Troubles are often the tools by which God fashions us for better things.
—Henry Ward Beecher[1]

A mong the participants in academic bioethical debates, a central moral discourse concerning reproductive genetic technologies (RGTs) is the relief of suffering. The word suffering rarely appears in print, because it is a taken for granted value that does not even need to be said. And, of course, all the uses of RGTs are implicitly justified as relieving suffering of some sort—preventing cystic fibrosis avoids an early painful death for a child, making a child a regular height avoids the suffering of being short in a world where tall people have social advantages, and providing parents with a badly desired male child relieves the suffering of those parents.[2]

Indeed, this concern with the relief of suffering could be said to be one of the most central and deeply assumed themes in Western civilization. For example, public policy seems to be designed to make people suffer less through improving transit, healthcare, race relations, the food supply, employment, and so on. Just imagine announcing to friends that you do not want to decrease suffering in the world but to just keep it constant. You would be treated with contempt because the relief of suffering, and its cousin "progress," is one of the faiths of a secular civilization.[3] As others have said, if you want to know what is most important to a civilization, look at the relative height of the buildings. In medieval Europe the largest building was the cathedral. In many contemporary cities, it is the medical center, dedicated as it is to the relief of suffering.[4]

In this chapter, I begin by examining some academic writing about how medicine and science describe suffering to help us understand what is at stake here. I also closely examine writings about suffering in Christianity where suffering has meaning and does not necessarily need to be eradicated in all cases. I find that there is a particular discourse about meaningful suffering that is used to oppose RGTs, and I separately analyze the pro-lifers and non–pro-lifers who use it.

The Medical Discourse of Suffering

The term "suffering" is used vaguely in discussions of medicine and RGTs; therefore, more precision is helpful. Eric Cassell, focusing on suffering in medicine, defines suffering as "the state of severe distress associated with events that threaten the intactness of a person."[5] Similar to other scholars, Cassell makes a critical distinction between "pain" and "suffering."[6] Pain can lead to suffering—that threat to personal intactness—but not necessarily. For example, while the pain of cancer can cause suffering, many women consider the pain of childbirth to not be suffering, because it is not a threat to their personal intactness. Moreover, Cassell demonstrates that people suffer, as defined above, even though they are not in pain. As another example, consider the threat to personal intactness (suffering) a disease in a child causes *for the parents*. Most parents consider it part of being parents to protect their child from pain and to have their children prosper. While not having the physical pain of their children, most parents suffer because their personal identity as parents is threatened, and to love their children is part of their self. They would not suffer if they did not care about their children.

As many scholars have noted, we live in a society where medicine is no longer simply supposed to relieve or avoid pain but also to relieve suffering, a process called the medicalization of suffering.[7] For example, Prozac and Ritalin do not relieve pain, but rather relieve suffering. Another example comes from the World Health Organization, which famously defined the task of medicine in a radically expansionist manner: "Health is a state of complete physical, mental, and social well-being and not merely the absence of disease or infirmity."[8] Campbell summarizes this trend in the treatment of suffering by arguing that "we live in a medical and moral culture that seeks to banish the experience of suffering from the human condition. . . . Suffering, in the ideology of contemporary medicine, is an evil, a fate worse than death; and it is perhaps an unmitigated evil, whose presence in human experience is a symbol of failure, and thus is not to be tolerated but conquered through technology."[9] This is what I will call the medical discourse of suffering.

RGTs are useful for the elimination of pain, suffering, or both. Using preimplantation genetic diagnosis to avoid having a child with cystic fibrosis could be justified as an attempt to reduce both the literal pain that a child would experience, as well as the suffering of that child and the family. Other objectives of RGTs are less about avoiding pain and more about avoiding suffering. Using RGTs to avoid producing a baby that would have early-onset Alzheimer's disease is not about eliminating pain, but rather the suffering that is associated with this disease. Using RGTs to make a baby more intelligent would be justified by arguing that this would eliminate the suffering the child would face for not being one of the best. (The actual "suffering" is probably that of the parents, whose "personal intactness" involves producing only the "best" children.)

Alternative Religious Discourses about Suffering

In the medical discourse of suffering, suffering has no meaning or purpose and should be eradicated through medicine. In contrast, in many religious traditions suffering has explicit meaning. Theologian Stanley Hauerwas even goes so far as to say that "the most decisive challenge which medicine raises for Christian convictions and morality involves the attempt to make suffering pointless and thus subject to elimination."[10]

The first and most obvious observation about religion and suffering is, according to Campbell, that "the experience of suffering is central to spirituality and the self-understanding of most religious communities."[11] For example, it could be argued that one of the central narratives in Christianity is that Christ suffered on the cross as substitutionary atonement for the sins of humanity. Similarly, Jews suffered under Pharaoh before the Exodus, and there have undoubtedly been many thousands of pages written about the book of Job in the Jewish and Christian traditions—Job being a person who suffered greatly at the hand of God. In sum, although there are vast and complicated discourses in (at least) the Jewish and Christian traditions regarding suffering, these discourses do not match the dominant medical discourse of suffering, and these religious discourses may be used by the respondents to talk about RGTs.

If the medical discourse is that suffering is meaningless, what possible meaning could suffering have for Christians? David H. Smith, building on the work of philosopher of religion John Hick, identifies three streams of discourse on suffering in the Christian tradition. The first discourse, labeled the Augustinian tradition, also was followed by the medieval church and Saint Thomas Aquinas, as well as later by Martin Luther, John Calvin and much later by theologians such as Karl Barth. Evil—and thus suffering—is the result of the Fall of man, which occurred when Adam and Eve were ejected from the Garden of Eden, leaving their perfect nature behind. The subsequent fallen nature of humanity not only inevitably suffers but also collectively deserves suffering as punishment for the original sin. Therefore, to try to eliminate all suffering is folly, because suffering is an ongoing punishment for original sin. Smith nicely points out that this view fits best in traditions that view God as a judge who "treats his human subjects according to their deserts" in a "fundamentally juridical" manner.[12] Christians using this particular version of a meaningful suffering discourse would not be interested in ending suffering that seemed to be willed by God.

A second discourse can be traced back to debates about the nature of the Trinity in the fourth century, which were largely debates about the nature of God. In short, the victorious group at the Council of Nicea was able to establish that the Son and the Father were of the same identity; thus, since Jesus suffered on the cross, God also suffers. Therefore, God "suffers with us; we do not suffer alone." Smith concludes that Christian art and literature throughout the ages—to say nothing of the movie *The Passion* by Mel Gibson a few years ago—"dwell on the suffering Christ because it was comforting." In the suffering of the believer, the believer is identified with God: "God himself suffers, precisely as you do."[13]

This particular discourse of suffering has three implications for arguments about relieving suffering. First, this discourse implies that "the optimal response to suffering" is not to stop it (which God would presumably be capable of doing), but rather to "suffer through" it, like God does. Since God does not end God's own suffering, then why should humans? Second, since suffering is accepted by God, this "suggests that suffering is eternal, unlikely to disappear." For those church members swimming in this stream of the theological river, trying to unequivocally end suffering would nearly be tantamount to denying the importance of God. Finally, people who argue that God suffers with us humans will be likely to "identify with the sufferings of others" because "this is the cause of God." This would generate a strong compassionate response to suffering, but not necessarily the desire to end suffering.[14]

A third discourse, which Smith labels the Irenaean tradition, was later adopted by liberal theologians of the eighteenth and nineteenth centuries such as Friedrich Schleiermacher. In this view, the Fall is less important, but rather, according to Genesis, human nature is at present imperfect. Humans are made in God's image, but, crucially, they must "perfect themselves as moral agents in order to live in God's likeness." Therefore, "evil is necessary as an obstacle to be overcome." Suffering is then "fundamentally pedagogical," and suffering leads to personal growth toward being more in God's likeness. Suffering then has a character forming or pedagogical quality; therefore, suffering should not be eradicated.[15]

While the Christian tradition talks about the meaningfulness of suffering, the Jewish tradition lacks a strong discourse about the positive value of suffering, particularly suffering from disease. As most primers on Jewish bioethics begin with some variation on "the mandate to heal," it is clear that in Judaism there is a strong commandment to heal disease and suffering.[16] For example, J. David Bleich claims that "the value with which human life is regarded in the Jewish tradition is maximized far beyond the value placed upon human life in the Christian tradition . . . the obligation to preserve life is commensurately all-encompassing."[17] The Jews interviewed for this project saw no value in suffering, and almost all seemed to look at RGTs through the lens of relieving suffering, which many perceived to be the divine mandate of *tikkun olam*, a religious requirement to heal or repair the world.

Using the Medical Discourse: The Meaninglessness of Suffering

Among the interviewees, almost everyone wanted to eliminate at least some genetic diseases, and nobody was in favor of all suffering. Even the people opposed to all RGTs would like to eliminate cystic fibrosis through what they considered to be "medicine," as long as it did not involve reproduction. That is, almost no one articulated an extreme Augustinian position, that *suffering* was deserved or part of God's will, and everyone used the medical discourse of suffering for some situations.

There were two general types of respondents—those who use both the medical discourse of suffering and a meaningful suffering discourse and those who use the medical discourse of suffering alone. The first group struggles to decide which discourse of suffering fits the new situation and often applies the meaningful suffering discourse. The second group only uses the medical discourse of suffering, and this group is most easily identified by their incredulous responses to follow up questions asking for an explanation for why they want to relieve someone of a disease that would lead to suffering.

For example, like many with whom we spoke, Tracy articulated an anguished pro-choice position on abortion when we discussed amniocentesis. He would want to know

> at the point we can abort the child, if we choose to do that. Not that we would, but at least it opens that possibility. And then having done that, then my wife, the mother of the child—we'd have to sit down and make some personal decisions because whatever we decide, we're going to have to live with it. And that means, you know, our conscience, you know, whatever guilt that attaches itself. We have to think about the child, because we're making a decision that's going to impact a third person. So, you know, you've got to take that child's—I don't want to call it rights, but you have to consider the impact on that child. Because essentially, I mean—and I'm not an antiabortionist. . . . I mean, if you're taking that child in the first trimester—you're still killing the child. I mean, it's—you know, that's just societal question about the right or wrong in that. But, that is a fact and let's put it this way—if you didn't intervene, the child would be born—all things being equal. . . . Then, you ask yourself, is thirty years of living the last part of which is going to be, not positive, but, the first part of which will be? Does that balance out? There's some tough questions here. You have—you literally have the life of this child in your hands. . . . My tendency would be that we would probably, if we could get the amniocentesis done at an early point, when we could determine early on during the first month of pregnancy that we would probably abort.

When we told him that with amniocentesis the abortion would not occur until much later than the first month of pregnancy, he was disturbed, but said:

> Still the tendency would be to abort because I know this disease. It's a miserable way to go; I mean this is not a pleasant thing. And by letting this child live and—I'm not mincing words here, cause that's what we're doing—I'm not talking about being born—we're letting it live. You've doomed it to an agonizing end.

Clearly he is not using the embryonic life discourse, but like many Americans, he has a developmental version of when the fetus becomes a person. As we would expect, his immediate response to preimplantation genetic diagnosis, which only destroys embryos, is positive:

TRACY: That's awesome. I mean that's a problem solver right there.

INTERVIEWER: Okay, so my question is, should they use this way of making . . .

TRACY: Absolutely. I mean, absolutely. I mean—you can't—you know that—isn't that called a blastocyst? Eight cells?

INTERVIEWER: Yes.

TRACY: [. . .]it's just a tissue mess. Yeah, sure, absolutely. I mean, that's the way to go. If they've got that technology, that would be awesome or if that's where this is headed to try and get there.

To explain further his motivation, he says:

You have this image of this child, dying in agony and the suffering that it has to go through and you have that option which is a possibility and then you have the option of not even risking that. It's not even a question. Of course. Why—you know, I'm not going to have a child go through that. You know, just to make some kind of philosophical point. That's crap.

He obviously does not think highly of the embryonic life discourse, which he considers to be a "philosophical point" that is "crap" when compared to relieving the suffering of cystic fibrosis.

Having stated his primary discourse, Tracy continues when queried about pre-implantation genetic diagnosis for early onset Alzheimer's disease that "ethically, it's still the same question and I have no objection to it. In terms of the severity of the decision, however, it's lower on the scale." For Tracy, preimplantation genetic diagnosis for deafness is "pretty far down the list, but as an ethical point—no, they're the same. I mean, if you can eliminate that possibility, yeah."

Later, after opposing preimplantation genetic diagnosis for obesity, Tracy clearly states that his decision-making about which RGTs are acceptable is based on whether they fit with his desire to eliminate anything he considers to be suffering. He says, "If you're trying to save that child from death or suffering, that's one thing, but if you're trying to give a child an advantage socially, without the child having any input into it, I think that's wrong." When discussing preimplantation genetic diagnosis for intelligence, he repeats that "again, it's not a life-saving situation and it doesn't avoid suffering." Like others we discussed in chapter 4, he turns to the secular discourse of nature, saying, "You know, there's a natural order of things, you know natural selection and, you know, it works." He turns to the social dignity/equality discourse with a Nazi analogy when he worries that in letting people select for intelligence "pretty soon you're at the point where you're deciding who's fit and we stuff ovens full of people who are found to be unfit."

Tracy's use of the medical discourse on suffering is very clear when he seemingly contradicts himself when he says he does not "want to have society in a position to decide who's fit and who's not fit to survive." While this sounds contradictory because he advocates deciding that people with certain diseases should not exist, this principle does not apply to conditions he defines as producing suffering, like cystic fibrosis. He is referring to other reasons that people use RGTs, such as to avoid having children with Down's syndrome. When asked to explain his statement about not wanting to have society decide who survives, he retorts:

> You go ask any parent of a child with Down's syndrome that question. At face value that child would be found unfit genetic anomaly, it's going to die, premature, it's retarded looks funny. Let's get rid of it. But everybody if you talk to almost every parent you talk to—had Down's kids; they're wonderful children and they're happy, they have almost an idyllic existence because they retain their innocence even to the point of death. Is that a bad thing? Should we eliminate those folks just cause they're different and they don't meet our norm? I don't think anybody should be in that position. And I certainly don't think as a culture, we should ever do that.

In short, people with Down's syndrome do not suffer, in his view, so they should be protected.

As the interview progresses, Tracy states that he is opposed to sex selection through any method, because a specific sex does not lead to suffering. When our conversation turns to human genetic engineering for cystic fibrosis, he again sees this as not even a legitimate question, responding, "Absolutely. I think they have an obligation to do it. . . . You kidding me— if you could eliminate one generation cystic fibrosis from the face of the planet, wouldn't you do it? Yeah, it's not even a question, of course." He then maintains the same distinctions with applications of human genetic engineering that he used when the technology under discussion was preimplantation genetic diagnosis. After we finished discussing the scenarios and turned to a follow-up question asking why we should eliminate disease, he summarized his discourse on suffering nicely:

> Some of these diseases—they're just pure agony. I mean people suffer. I don't think people should suffer when we have the ability to prohibit that from happening. And it's in the suffering and there's no societal gain in, you know, allowing diseases to run rampant. But, equally, I mean, there's no logical reason to stop them other than we have the obligation to prevent suffering, like all of us—in one way or the other.

Tracy has no question in his mind that what he defines as suffering is to be eliminated. He says at various points that it is an obligation and considers discourses that would oppose this position—like the embryonic life discourse—to be "crap."

Similarly, Allen also sees the relief of suffering as an unquestioned virtue. Like most others who did not also use a meaningful suffering discourse, Allen deeply assumes the medical discourse on suffering, and that the interviewer assumes that this discourse will fit with RGT applications that are diseases, that he does not explicitly say he wants to relieve suffering. It remains implicit.

Like many who were pro-choice on abortion, Allen also was reluctant to even talk in a way that seemed to impose his values on the hypothetical couple, saying of amniocentesis for cystic fibrosis, "I don't know. It's up to them. I think if it were me, and I probably—if I knew for sure that the child had cystic fibrosis, I don't know. I would be leaning probably towards an abortion, but if the wife wanted to have it, I would say, you know, to have it anyway."

He was enthusiastic about preimplantation genetic diagnosis, saying, "Well, I don't see why not. If they have a way of knowing, I don't see why they wouldn't do it. It's not harming anything. . . . because she's not—she's not pregnant." For early-onset Alzheimer's disease, he sees it as the same, saying, "They're still trying to stay away from a disease." The same for deafness. Avoiding disease is implicitly relieving suffering for people in this group. He did not think that there would be a need for preimplantation genetic diagnosis for obesity because "obesity is something that people can control, [so] I don't think that's enough reason to do that." Allen shows us his line between suffering and nonsuffering, saying, "I don't think it's anything serious enough to go through that procedure. I think it's something that—it's not any big deal for somebody to be obese, I don't think,—as opposed to being deaf or getting Alzheimer's when you're fifty. I mean I don't think obesity is in the same category as that."

For preimplantation genetic diagnosis for intelligence, he does not come up with the discourses we see in the previous chapters, but rather that lack of intelligence does not produce enough suffering. He says, "Well, I'm back to the same reasoning . . . I just don't think it's a good enough reason to alter—to make any alterations there."

He was in favor of sex selection abortion, and even more enthusiastic about preimplantation genetic diagnosis for sex selection and very in favor of sperm sorting, with this underlying degree of enthusiasm tied to avoiding destroying embryos or fetuses. However, for Allen, this has nothing to do with embryonic life, but rather has to do with the psychological suffering for the couple, saying the latter technologies are "less intrusive." When the conversation turned to human genetic engineering for cystic fibrosis, after describing the scenario and hypothetical couple to him, we asked:

INTERVIEWER: Do you think that they should do this?
ALLEN: Yes.
INTERVIEWER: Do you have any concerns about this technology at all?
ALLEN: No.

He does not need to justify his response. When asked after the scenarios had been described why we would want to stop people from getting genetic diseases, he responds: "So we could live—so we could live. Am I missing the question there?"

Almost everyone is opposed to some enhancements, even if it is only reproductive cloning. The medical suffering discourse operates in the negative as a discourse of opposition for the (relative) supporters of RGTs who only oppose enhancements. When an application is perceived as no longer reducing suffering, then it is wrong on those grounds. People who start by talking about eradicating suffering start debating with themselves part way through the interview about whether deaf or obese people suffer, or whether early-onset Alzheimer's disease results in suffering. They eventually conclude that people who lack super strength or enhanced intelligence do not suffer and say so in their disapproval.

Although not always explicitly articulated, I believe that all Americans use this discourse at some point in their lives. Every person has had a disease, however transitory, and everyone has used the discourse of eliminating suffering to talk about a cold or some worse disease. The question

I began this research project with was as follows: In which new situations that they encounter will they use this discourse because the situation is "the same?" If I were to have asked about healing a newly emergent form of cancer in adults, I expect that people would almost universally to see this new situation as "the same" as previous situations where the medical discourse of suffering was used, and thus say, "Yes, of course, heal that disease and relieve that suffering." But, is the salient feature of the situation of using preimplantation genetic diagnosis to eliminate cystic fibrosis "just like" previous situations of relieving the suffering of disease, or is it "just like" other instances of "killing innocent persons," "letting God do what God is going to do," or "respecting the dignity and equality of other persons?" For the people we just discussed, it is often "just like" other instances of healing disease.

The discourse of the relief of suffering is ubiquitous in contemporary society—just think of pharmaceutical advertising alone. It is then always primed and then ready to be applied to new situations that people encounter. If an RGT is perceived by the respondent to relieve suffering, then it requires the availability of other discourses to not use the medical discourse of suffering. In the previous chapters we have seen these powerful alternative discourses that people use to essentially say, "Yes, cystic fibrosis would result in suffering, but that RGT would either destroy embryonic life, trespass into God's realm, or require treating people unequally." There remains one final alternative discourse to the medical discourse of suffering that I have not yet presented—that suffering is meaningful and should therefore not be eradicated.

Meaningful Suffering

While everyone has the medical discourse of suffering available, some people have another discourse of suffering that they apply to some new situations. In my theoretical framework, this discourse has been used in previous situations where the suffering has been beneficial, and these people are primed to look for new situations of potentially meaningful suffering in RGTs. What this results in is that people who use the meaningful suffering discourse see many of the borderline cases (e.g., preimplantation genetic diagnosis for deafness or obesity) as meaningful suffering, whereas people who lack this discourse are more likely to see this as meaningless suffering and use the medical discourse. The survey demonstrates this by showing that people who use the discourse of meaningful suffering are opposed to more applications of RGTs than those who do not use this discourse.[18] More specifically, the in-depth interviews show that the specific meaning of suffering for those who do and do not use the embryonic life discourse is the third discourse identified by Smith, the Irenaean, where suffering is meaningful because it is pedagogical for the sufferer or for those around the sufferer.

Meaningful Suffering among the Pro-lifers

As shown in table 3 in chapter 3, 87 percent of the pro-lifer, strong opponents of RGTs in the survey who regularly attend religious services use the meaningful suffering discourse. Thus, they use these discourses at some point, but when exactly? In the in-depth interviews, interviewees often start with intertwining the two discourses when discussing technologies that potentially harm embryos, and then continue with the meaningful suffering discourse to justify opposing an RGT when embryos are not at risk.

For example, Jack is a fundamentalist. He thinks with amniocentesis that the hypothetical couple should "accept the outcome as it is without testing." In regards to preimplantation genetic diagnosis, Jack says:

> I don't see a problem with in vitro fertilization for couples who are otherwise infertile as far as using that as a method to get pregnant or to have a child of their own. The part of the problem that I have with that are the leftover fertilized eggs, okay? If that were me personally, . . . what I would want to make sure is that these eggs, fertilized eggs, that weren't used, because they don't use them all, [are used.]

He continues using the embryonic life discourse, saying, "I believe that the fertilized egg is life. As a matter of fact, the people who basically engineer these, the geneticists or doctors, consider them life too because they keep them frozen otherwise they would die. . . . So that's kind of how I feel about in vitro fertilization. So it's okay as long as the [fertilized] eggs are not destroyed because that, in my opinion, is life."

He follows up this statement with a combination of the embryonic life, individual dignity/equality, and meaningful suffering discourses:

> The fertilized egg is life, diseased or not. There are certainly purposes for people; I mean there are people born with birth defects all the time. I don't have

any personal friends that have children with Down syndrome or anything like that but from what I know, I mean, I'm an acquaintance to certain people . . . who have a Down's child and this child is now an adult, still lives at home and is pretty much one of the most loving people around and there is certainly something worthwhile that that person can give others. So birth defects are not— there is still something, a relationship that can be had with someone with cystic fibrosis or whatever the birth defect may be. There can be a purpose there, I believe.

Jack says the presence of this child with Down's syndrome has been pedagogical for others—he can "give to others." As the interview continues, he interweaves the Promethean fatalist, individual dignity/equality, and embryonic life discourses. For example, he is opposed to sperm sorting because "you take the chance out of what God would have for you by doing it that way."

When the interview turns to human genetic engineering for cystic fibrosis, he says he does not

see a problem with that. I mean, that's eradicating disease. I think we've eradicated small pox except for the vials that are still in some lab somewhere unfortunately. But you know, diseases can be eradicated and it's a medical procedure. And there's no harm to the fetus and no possibility of another fertilized egg or fetus being aborted. I don't know how far away that really is but I mean, they do in vitro and in utero surgery already.

Like other conservative Protestants who say that the answers to contemporary questions can be found in the Bible, Jack says that he "would hold it up to a witness test as to what the Bible says" and concludes that the Bible would support human genetic engineering for cystic fibrosis. However, in the situation of human genetic engineering for deafness, he returns to arguing that people who may be suffering benefit others:

It's difficult because I think of deaf people who have had very good gifts to offer like Beethoven, Helen Keller; they have had . . . They took what they had and were able to develop their gifts regardless of the fact that they were deaf. Had they had hearing, would they have been able to give to society what they did? I don't know. I mean, I don't know the answer to that question. So that's more of a gray area for me as opposed to the others that we've talked about.

People who do not use the meaningful suffering discourse would tend to see this situation as meaningless suffering and thus argue for its eradication.

We later followed up by asking whether we want to stop people from getting genetic diseases. Jack said, "Again, I'm not so sure that it necessarily has to be stopped because there could certainly be blessings in good things as well as bad things and disease is certainly considered to be a bad thing." When later asked to describe in his own words what constitutes a disease, he further reveals his thinking about suffering, saying, "there can certainly be comfort found in disease or mishaps." The idea that there is comfort in disease or mishaps is again not an idea expressed by those who exclusively use the medical discourse of suffering. He clarifies himself further when we asked if we should eliminate all suffering, to which he responded:

> I would say not necessarily because again, there can be good means that comes out of suffering. Suffering, I mean, Paul says that suffering builds character and perseverance. . . . There certainly are some character-building things that can come out of suffering. Then you can help other people who maybe suffer from the same thing that you suffered through five years ago. Now they're suffering from it but because you've been through it, you can better empathize or sympathize and help them get through whatever it is the affliction might be.

Most of the people who used the meaningful suffering discourse switched to one of the other strongly oppositional discourses in regards to the applications of RGTs that could not be portrayed as reducing suffering. For example, a lack of superintelligence, rectified by use of human genetic engineering, is hard to construe as relieving suffering. Jack switches to Promethean fatalism, which he had used at various places earlier in the interview, saying, "Again, you're playing too much of God in that and not allowing the child to be what that child could be or was meant to be by adjusting their intelligence." This continues with cloning, when he states, "I don't think that person is their own person or the person who they were taken from and God's already created that person. If He wanted that person to be the same then he would have created an identical twin."

Similarly, Peter, a retired bookkeeper who weekly attends his Catholic church, quickly displays all four of the discourses used by strong opponents under close examination in this book. When asked about abortion after amniocentesis, Peter says they should "not test the fetus and see what happens" because:

I think that whatever happens, the Lord designates that and it's His will, even if the child is born with cystic fibrosis. It's His will for that to happen for a reason we don't know. It may be that in caring for that child, the parents gain a lot of grace that will help them when they need it. . . . And I know of . . . [a girl],[19] totally helpless, and her parents have cared for her; struggled, cared . . . spent a lot of time and anguish caring for this child, it was their primary mission. Obviously when you do something like that there's no thanks . . . coming from the child or from anybody really and I think they build up their grace by doing that. So sometimes a child like that is a gift.

A child who has a disease, who is suffering, can be "a gift" for others. When next asked about preimplantation genetic diagnosis, he opposed destroying leftover embryos, saying, "That's life in its beginning. . . . We believe that life begins at conception, and that's all we've been taught, and I abide by that."

He opposes sperm sorting because it is "tampering with what nature intends." When we discuss human genetic engineering for cystic fibrosis, he says, "I can't give you a snap answer on that one. I would have to think about that one." He struggles to decide whether this situation fits best with previous situations where he has used the medical discourse of suffering or the meaningful suffering discourse. He says, "This somehow contradicts my previous statement about that person being a gift to the parents, but they already have two gifts so to speak [two other children with cystic fibrosis in our hypothetical scenario] and this would prevent it in ongoing generations." Put more simply, the parents are going to have enough pedagogical experience of suffering from the first two children, and since cystic fibrosis is not an absolute good, then perhaps it would be good to stop it. He brings the Promethean fatalist discourse back into his internal debate, saying, "I would have to think about that but then I have to go back to God's will. Maybe God's will is that this child should have this also for whatever reason we don't know. So this would be a conflict with me so I can't really give you a definite answer without really studying and contemplating both ends of this." He sees the other applications of human genetic engineering as "the same dilemma."

Meaningful Suffering among the Non–pro-lifers

Many non–pro-lifers—those who do not use the embryonic life discourse—also use the meaningful suffering discourse. A smaller subset of this group uses the meaningful suffering discourse to oppose abortion for

cystic fibrosis and most other RGTs, just like those on the other side of
the discursive divide, but without mentioning embryonic life. The larger
subset approves of abortion for cystic fibrosis and preimplantation genetic
diagnosis for health reasons using the medical discourse of suffering, but
shifts to the meaningful suffering discourse to oppose what they consider
to be enhancements. For example, Trudy is a Catholic nurse. She does not
use the embryonic life discourse during our interview, but she is one of
the respondents who opposes abortion by using only the other three oppositional discourses. At the mention of amniocentesis for cystic fibrosis,
she immediately states, "Just because the child has cystic fibrosis doesn't
mean that they're not a person of value and of worth and there's a whole
lot of worse things that can happen to you. And I've personally taken care
of kids with cystic fibrosis, and they're great kids and I don't think that
their families think that their lives have been lessened by having them in
it." Trudy is mixing the discourse of individual dignity/equality with the
discourse of meaningful suffering—the meaning being that others learn
from the sufferer.

She is opposed to preimplantation genetic diagnosis, saying, "At some
point, you have to have faith and let God be God. . . . If you can't trust
that whatever He gives you, you can handle, then you don't have any business having it in the first place. Any one of us could have a child with a
defect, or as soon as they're born, an accident happens and then you have
a crippled child or whatever . . . You take what you're given and you deal
with it because you'll be given the strength to deal with it." This is the
Promethean fatalist discourse, and she uses the same discourse to oppose
other applications of preimplantation genetic diagnosis.

She continues by using a combination of the individual dignity/equality
and the meaningful suffering discourses. She tells a personal story:

I have a [relative] who . . . lost a baby due to a [serious health condition].[20] She
lived for two weeks and was in intensive care the whole time but it was a really
spiritual and emotionally uplifting time for our whole family and I wouldn't
trade [her] two weeks on earth for . . . heck a lot of people's ninety years. She
did a lot in her two weeks and they knew before she was born there was going
to be a problem, could they have aborted her? Yeah, I guess they could have . . .
I mean they wouldn't have, but people have opted to do that, but they would
have missed out on a hugely rewarding experience even though she only lived
for two weeks, it was a good two weeks. It was not just a good two weeks for
her but for everybody around her. Even the nurses down at [the hospital] said

this is just amazing, it was really cool and I wouldn't trade that experience for anything. And I think whenever we start saying this suffering or that suffering, so what, life is full of suffering. And it's how we handle it and how we trust in it and how we have a better life.

Again, Trudy is not in favor of suffering itself—she is, after all, a nurse. But, in this discourse, she is saying the relief of suffering is not paramount because suffering can be a pedagogical experience for those around the sufferer. Later, she talked about her own family using the meaningful suffering discourse, saying:

> We've been blessed by not having genetic diseases [but] we have a kid with severe [disease] and one with [less severe disease] . . . which certainly can be crippling. But I wouldn't . . . shoot, I wouldn't change them for the world. No, I think that's a unique challenge. . . . You know I think that lives are enriched by dealing with adversity. . . . You'd be cutting out a lot of great kids, if you just said no. . . . Some of the best kids in the world are Down's syndrome.

She later elaborated that suffering:

> can be good and in our society we tend to think of it as just bad, and that we need to do away with suffering. I think a lot of growth comes from suffering and you can't . . . to alleviate that would alleviate growth and so you can't, just getting rid of it, that's not the point. . . . But in the end, no I don't think suffering is bad. I think suffering can be good. I think it makes you stronger and certainly develops the faith.

Later, when we get to human genetic engineering for cystic fibrosis, Trudy says that "On principle no [but] that would be a harder call. I would certainly sympathize with where they're at, they're already living through it and then they have the opportunity to have a child without it . . . that would be a hard call," she continues, but "I would still say no. It's still the same thing."

When asked why she seems equivocal about human genetic engineering for cystic fibrosis but is steadfastly opposed to preimplantation genetic diagnosis for cystic fibrosis, Trudy invokes the individual dignity/equality discourse again, saying, that with preimplantation genetic diagnosis, "You're throwing out what you think is defective. I mean there you're just saying you're not good, you're not good and you're basically not given a life a chance because it's not good. Here you're not doing that . . . you're altering it." Altering instead of picking is what makes the analogy with individual dignity/equality inoperative for human genetic engineering for cystic fibrosis.

Note that Trudy does not appear to be opposed to destroying embryos per se, but only to deciding which to destroy based on their characteristics. She also mentioned in an aside that embryonic stem cell research is "not real black and white in my mind." Her not using the embryonic life discourse, which she clearly is familiar with, may be due to what she sees as the degree of independence she has from the teachings of the Catholic Church. At a later point, talking about modifying embryos to avoid disease, she states, "I'm not sure what the church's stand is on that, I'm not sure the church knows what the church's stand is on that, but because in genetics all of that is wrong. But some of that, the fine tuning of it, how can it be wrong? . . . In some instances, that might not be so bad." Despite being a bit tortured on human genetic engineering for cystic fibrosis, when we turn to what she considers to be human genetic engineering for enhancements, like obesity and intelligence, she is brief and unequivocal: "No that's totally wrong." As for cloning, that is "just ridiculous."

This discourse of meaningful suffering is also used by those who are supportive of abortion and of using RGTs that destroy embryos or fetuses, suggesting a moderately porous divide. For example, Irene, a mainline Protestant woman in her mid-fifties, is ambivalent about suffering, but clearly does not hold it to be the ultimate enemy when discussing amniocentesis for cystic fibrosis:

> I mean first [of] all it's not my place to make their decision but I certainly would have no problems with anybody going ahead and doing everything that science can do to prevent a baby born with a disease that we have the power to do something about. I certainly wouldn't abort a pregnancy based on a one-in-four chance of something being wrong and I wouldn't automatically say about cystic fibrosis "that's a terrible thing. If the genetic tests show that the baby has it, abort it." I mean, that would be a long and hard decision for me to make if it were my personal situation. I don't know enough about the disease to know what the quality of life for the child is, but I think every child is born with capabilities so I would have to get a lot more information if it were happening to me. But I would be supportive in that circumstance of a couple making that decision. I mean that's a terrible decision to have to make.

She later concludes that "an abortion is not the worst thing that can happen." Like many mainline Protestants she is conflicted and clearly has a developmental concept of when the fetus becomes a person:

> It's not something that I would say "every woman has a right to her own body up until, you know, whatever." I can't be that liberal in my attitudes. I believe life is sacred and up to a certain point maybe the mother's circumstances and the circumstances of that pregnancy outweigh that baby's right. I can't really think of things as being a fetus versus a baby. To me that pregnancy . . . I mean in my mind that's a . . . that's a child. And there . . . there may be moral . . . grey areas at first but boy, once that baby is fully formed and you know it's moving in you, to me that . . . that means that the baby has equal rights if not . . . you know they just can't be . . . can't be ignored. . . . I can't go so far as to say that the loss of that child is a murder until it's born. So I'm . . . you know . . . I'm . . . I'm a mixture of . . . I'm a mess.

Given her developmental notion of when the fetus becomes a person and clearly lacking the embryonic life discourse, Irene responds to preimplantation genetic diagnosis for cystic fibrosis by saying that the technology is "God's gift. If we have the technology to do something like that I think that's wonderful." She is profoundly ambivalent about using preimplantation genetic diagnosis for early-onset Alzheimer's disease, saying that "the need to have Gap children is kind of pathetic." She initially opposes sex selection by any means using the same discourse of opposition to the perfection of children, but later uses the secular nature discourse, saying:

> We don't always make wise choices and there are reasons after so many millions of years for humans to be the way they are and it's just . . . you know that old commercial about Mother . . . don't . . . don't . . . what was the phrase about Mother Nature? Don't mess with Mother Nature.

When it comes to the alternative technology of human genetic engineering instead of preimplantation genetic diagnosis, Irene has no particular concerns, but reiterates her previous criteria of acceptability. For "something awful" like cystic fibrosis, then the technology is good; for something that is like a "designer baby" to satisfy the cultural needs of parents, then it is unacceptable. Later, she discussed why she wants to stop children from getting some genetic diseases and in her response it becomes clear why people who use the meaningful suffering discourse approve of fewer applications of RGTs:

> [We have] close friends of the family [who have] a daughter with degenerative muscular dystrophy. . . . Watching her struggle . . . if there were a way to have prevented that and still have Julia as Julia, you know I just . . . how wonderful that would have been to have been able to detect that gene and remove that from her and leave that girl intact. I mean it's just such a tragedy to see a human being have to deal with what she knows is a degenerative disease and, she's now wheelchair bound and will continue to get worse. And what's ahead of her is just nothing . . . you know it's awful to think. . . . I will also say, and this may sound strange, but for a family to deal with a genetic illness like that, I think can also be a . . . growth experience for that family. I don't think it's the end of the world to have a child with a debilitating disease because parents rise to the occasion and they become more than they might have even know they could become dealing with it. So, I don't think it's the end of the world. . . . But, wow, what that family has been through. And how they have risen to those needs. It just . . . it's . . . it's just an inspiration.

Irene is in favor of many applications of RGTs. Her enthusiasm, her drive, for the new technologies are a bit less than those who exclusively use the medical discourse. I would argue that this is because she has used this discourse of the meaningful suffering in the past and sees it as analogous to at least some instances of RGTs.

Similarly, Beatrice is a liberal Protestant in her sixties. Like many liberal Protestants, she is pro-choice on abortion. When asked about what a hypothetical couple who are carriers of cystic fibrosis should do, she anticipates the next question in the interview by saying they should either adopt or "conceive and then have some genetic testing and decide at that point whether the child has [the cystic fibrosis genes] and then opt to abort. But I wouldn't want to have to go through that decision. . . . If they decided to do it I would support them."

Abortion in this case would eliminate suffering, roughly along the lines of the medical discourse. Abortion, for Beatrice, would be, as she states, "A traumatic and emotional experience, I guess for the parents." She also mentions as important the "strain between two people" caused by having a child with cystic fibrosis and says, "Just knowing the burdens of a chronic illness from all of the realms that I've talking about financially, and emotionally, and just thinking that's going on all your life would be very difficult."

Beatrice simply says "yes" to preimplantation genetic diagnosis for cystic fibrosis, saying, "It just feels better to me that you wouldn't have to make the decision about aborting. For me, it would be a lot less emotional? . . . this is conceived out here. It's not really, I don't think, quite yet a part of you. Even though it is a part of you, I don't feel like it's yet a part of me until it would be implanted. I like that option a lot better." Beatrice clearly does not use the embryonic life discourse, and preimplantation genetic diagnosis would relieve the suffering of the woman, compared to having an abortion.

Beatrice approves of preimplantation genetic diagnosis for early-onset Alzheimer's disease and deafness. She says deafness is worse because of differential suffering. For deafness, again the deeply assumed medical discourse emerges. She says, that deafness "will be a handicap they would have for their entire life and maybe that's the difference. A child with cystic fibrosis and a deaf child would have that all of their life; whereas, someone predisposed to Alzheimer's disease would still have, hopefully, some part of their life without disease. Who knows? They might not even live to the time where. . . . They might be dead from another disease. Maybe the factor is that it's a permanent, lifelong handicap."

She is opposed to preimplantation genetic diagnosis for obesity because you could control that on your own as an adult by eating less. At preimplantation genetic diagnosis for intelligence, she abandons the medical discourse of suffering and turns to the meaningful suffering discourse. She begins with the Promethean fatalist discourse, saying, "I just don't think God would want humans to decide about every single thing." She continues, "I think it's grace how you are defined once you're born. And, in a sense, if everybody was [intelligent] . . . we'd be like little robots. No one would have any challenges. I don't think you can grow unless you have some challenges, pain, or maybe not suffering, but if you don't have those, you can't grow." She is not willing to call not being genetically engineered as superintelligent "suffering," but she makes the general point that "challenges" have a pedagogical use and should not necessarily be eradicated.

She is opposed to sex selection, eventually using the Promethean fatalist discourse, saying, "I want to say that it is the spirit, a higher being, God, who would choose which one." She is in favor of human genetic engineering for cystic fibrosis and describes the boundaries of the health promotion domain where it resides, saying, "I guess that scenario doesn't feel any different than the ones previous, whether you're testing for cystic fibrosis, whatever way they're testing. It seems more like a procedure or an operation, or any other type of treatment for an illness." Because it is a "procedure or an operation," like previous situations of health promotion, she uses the medical discourse.

For human genetic engineering for other conditions, Beatrice opposes these by using the same arguments that she used earlier. By the time we finish with cloning, she uses the individual dignity/equality discourse and says, "I feel like they're treating life, or someone's, their child, as an object, or as a materialistic type thing they can choose and buy and make all the decisions about. . . . Something that you might not like it if it's a certain way, but it's okay if it's successful and smart, male or female. So, yeah. I don't think they should be able to do that."

We later asked about eliminating all of people's suffering, and she clarified her use of the meaningful suffering discourse by saying that suffering "makes us stronger people, in order to see others' suffering. And that suffering that others have may be different, their suffering may not even be as bad as someone else's or might be better. It's all relative, but I think people grow in that way, society as people. I think without it, we wouldn't be caring people."

Those with the more permissive line between health and enhancements (e.g., stopping at improving intelligence) use the medical discourse of suffering to proclaim that this is not suffering. Those with the less permissive line (e.g., stopping at marginal diseases such as deafness) often use the same meaningful suffering discourse as do the strongest opponents of RGTs. In the survey, 77 percent of non–pro-lifer (relative) proponents of RGTs *do* use the meaningful suffering discourse to oppose at least some RGTs.[21] This suggests that there is not a strong discursive divide between the two sides of the abortion debate, or between the strong opponents and (relative) proponents of RGTs.

The Social Location of Suffering Discourses

It is clear that these discourses of suffering are not equally used in each religious tradition. The people with whom we spoke can be split into three groups when it comes to talking about relieving suffering through RGTs. The first group, largely dominated by the nonreligious, Jews, and liberal Catholics, only use the medical discourse about suffering and not the meaningful suffering discourse. These respondents cannot see another side to the debate and, when asked about whether we should use RGTs to alleviate genetic disease, do not even understand why anyone would even ask the question. This is also the most permissive group when it comes to RGT interventions. While they will oppose some enhancements, they generally do not do so by claiming that any resulting suffering is meaningful.

The second group, a mix of mainline Protestants, Jews, and Catholics, is not incredulous at the thought of not relieving the suffering of disease and understands why there might be a debate, but, in the end, they quite clearly fall on the side of relieving suffering through RGTs. They will use the meaningful suffering discourse to oppose enhancements. The third group of in-depth interviewees with whom we spoke, largely conservative Protestants (evangelicals and fundamentalists), tended to see a legitimate debate about whether we should end suffering through RGTs and were more likely to conclude that suffering has pedagogical value in developing either character or empathy (e.g., in theological terms, to grow into God's likeness). The survey shows similar results.[22]

To speculate about why conservative Protestants would be the most likely to use this discourse, we can start by repeating that suffering is common theme in the Christian tradition. Often these discussions occur under the rubric of theodicy, which classically asks the question, how can evil (and thus suffering) exist in the world if there is indeed an omniscient, omnipotent, and benevolent God? Note that there is only a theodicy if God is indeed omniscient and omnipotent, yet we have seen in chapter 4 that it is only the conservative Protestants and traditionalist Catholics who use the Promethean fatalist discourse, which presumes an omniscient and omnipotent God. This suggests that it is only members of these two groups that would face a theodicy and that the other religious groups' conception of God does not result in the theodicy problem.

There have been many solutions to the theodicy problem in the history of theology, and the academic descriptions of suffering in the Christian tradition are part of this debate. Each of the three discourses for how suffering can be meaningful could serve as a solution for those religious persons whose conceptions of God require a theodicy to be meaningful. Conservative Protestants and traditionalist Catholics are then the most likely to use the meaningful suffering discourse because they are also the ones who use a discourse of an omnipotent, omniscient God.

It remains an interesting question why the Irenean solution to theodicy, where suffering is pedagogical and through suffering we grow into God's likeness, is the one theodicy selected by these religious groups. This may be due to the fact that these religions are influenced by contemporary American culture.

Bill McKibben notes that three-quarters of Americans say in public opinion polls that the Bible teaches that "God helps those who help themselves." That is, he continues, "three out of four Americans believe that this uber-American idea, a notion at the core of our current individualist politics and culture, which was in fact uttered by Ben Franklin, actually appears in Holy Scripture."[23] This is an example of how people often elevate components of their culture to religious principle. Similarly, the idea that suffering exists and serves no productive purpose as the other religious meaningful suffering discourses imply is anathema to the American ethos. We are not to lie in our suffering, even if God were to be with us. Rather, we are to use our suffering to achieve new heights, to pull ourselves up by our bootstraps, and to live the American dream. This also explains the medical suffering discourse—we should not accept suffering, but strive to eradicate suffering. While these two discourses about suffering are used to support opposite conclusions in the RGT debate, they both seem to be a part of a deeper American culture.

Conclusion

Suffering is central to discussions of RGTs. The medical discourse of suffering, in which suffering has no meaning and should be eradicated, is used by nearly everyone with whom we spoke at least at some point. The only question is whether it was in competition with the alternative discourse of meaningful suffering, where suffering is pedagogical for either the person or the people surrounding that person. The meaningful suffering discourse is used by the stronger opponents of RGTs.

This section of the book also has been dedicated to evaluating whether a future RGT debate will be effective. Analogously to the previous two chapters, I find that the pro-lifers also use the meaningful suffering discourse to discuss not only abortion but also RGTs that do not implicate embryos. In chapters 4 and 5, I established Promethean fatalism and individual dignity/equality as part of the discursive framework for a broader issue domain called opposition to genetic control, which includes abortion and these RGTs; this chapter adds the final discourse of meaningful suffering to that framework. With these three discourses, we now see the boundaries of this distinct domain that includes both RGTs and abortion for cystic fibrosis, suggesting that these issues are already merged.

However, this merged issue domain will not create a discursive wall that would preclude conversations about RGTs. There is, of course, a group of non–pro-lifers who never describe suffering as meaningful and thus lack a shared discourse with opponents. However, as in previous chapters, the interviews show a group of non–pro-lifers who are opposed as the pro-lifers to the same RGTs, and using all the same discourses, except the embryonic life discourse that defines the supposed divide. This group then has a highly porous boundary across the abortion divide. Moreover, the larger group of the non–pro-lifers who use the meaningful suffering discourse do so to oppose enhancements. This moderately porous divide reveals a number of shared discourses with which to discuss at least a number of RGTs. As I conclude in the previous chapters, a significant number of non–pro-lifers can act as a communicative bridge with the pro-lifers in discussions about RGTs.

CHAPTER SEVEN

Will Religious Discourse about Reproductive Genetic Technologies Limit Debate?

We are placed into various life-spheres, each of which is governed by different laws. Religious ethics have settled with this fact in different ways.—Max Weber[1]

In the previous four chapters, I have examined not only which discourses religious people use to oppose reproductive genetic technologies (RGTs) but also whether a future debate would be limited by a lack of shared discourses across the abortion divide. In this chapter I separately evaluate the second reason people may not want to debate RGTs—that the debate will occur with explicitly religious discourse. Scholars have long been concerned that specifically religious discourse in the public sphere would have a particularly negative impact on willingness to deliberate.

This concern is reflected in Hunter's culture wars theory, which is based on other long-standing intellectual traditions. In this theory, the two sides of the culture war each have a "worldview," a hierarchical discursive structure where the most abstract and deeply assumed discourses are at the pinnacle. For example, what Hunter calls the orthodox worldview has at its pinnacle the discourse of "there is transcendent authority," meaning that there is a God whom we should consider when deciding how to behave. In the intellectual tradition that produces the worldview idea, each worldview is the equivalent of a religion—they contain the most deeply assumed "facts" about reality.[2] Specifically religious discourse, such as "God says in Psalm 139 that abortion is murder," points to the ultimate discourse.

What impacts deliberation is that in worldview theory, the worldviews are not only mutually exclusive and incompatible, but exposure to someone with another worldview results in a "certain desecration" of one's own worldview.[3] This is because the most abstract discourses in a worldview are so deeply assumed that they are one's sense of reality, and to encounter someone who does not share reality is deeply disturbing. Just like meeting mentally ill people who are in their own reality is disturbing to us, for someone with an orthodox worldview, meeting someone who does not unquestionably assume that "there is transcendent authority" is similarly threatening. This is why the most uncommon religions—those with very distinct worldviews which we often label "cults"—try to stop their members from interacting with people with other worldviews through social isolation.[4] Therefore, specifically religious discourse about RGTs will be particularly corrosive to deliberation because this religious discourse points to a person's ultimate assumptions about reality, which would threaten the ultimate reality of the discussion partner. Worldview theorists would then presume that people would avoid conversations where religious language is used.

Political theorists see the same problem with religious discourse in the public sphere. Their concerns are older than the founding of the United States, and they were certainly the motivation for liberal theorists such as John Locke, who strongly influenced the founders of this country. Indeed, the main lesson that Locke and his contemporaries learned from the Thirty Years' War in the early seventeenth century was that mixing religion and politics could lead to violence. A typical summary of this concern comes from Cynthia Cohen, who writes, "Liberal thought has tended to maintain that religion is too divisive to provide a constructive voice in public policy debates within democratic pluralistic societies. . . . Religious belief there is said to seriously threaten social stability."[5] Similarly, Gary Belkin, describing the history of bioethics, claims that liberal democratic theory "was attractive to many (including some early figures in the bioethics movement) for compelling reasons—to avoid civil war in a secular state over competing visions of what is 'moral'."[6]

The liberal theorists' solution is that people should use "public reason" in the public sphere—arguments that can be justified using discourse that everyone shares. As Robert Audi summarizes, "When there must be coercion, liberal democracies try to justify it in terms of considerations—such as public safety—that any rational adult citizen will find persuasive and can identify with."[7] For example, if society is going to ban cloning, it has to be for reasons that are intelligible to all. Making claims that are ultimately justified by using your particular religious tradition will not be intelligible to others and will discourage conversation, and therefore are not allowed. Note that many liberal theorists exclude not only religious discourse for this reason but also any "comprehensive doctrine" that is not universally shared, such as certain philosophies.[8] The culture wars literature and the political theory literature then would predict that people will not want to or be unable to have a conversation about RGTs if such a conversation uses religious discourse.

The Controversy over "God Talk" in the Public Sphere

The public does not seem to share the concerns of the theorists, and the frank religiosity of much public discourse in the United States makes it unusual among Western industrialized nations. " 'God talk' as much as 'rights talk' is the way Americans speak. American politics is indecipherable if severed from the panoply and interplay of America's religions," concludes social ethicist Jean Bethke Elshtain.[9] Yet, how much "God talk" should be allowed in public debate has been controversial from the birth of the nation. This level of "God talk" may well be a structural constraint on the health of the public sphere.

That "God talk" can be controversial beyond the substance of what is being said is clear by looking at two examples from the 2004 presidential election season. George W. Bush was, according to many "among the most openly religious presidents in U.S. history."[10] He said that Jesus is his favorite philosopher, he "prayed 'for the strength to do the Lord's will' in Iraq," and said, "I believe God wants me to be president."[11] In the 2003 State of the Union address, to explain why we will succeed in helping the needy, he said, "Yet there's power, wonder-working power, in the goodness and idealism and faith of the American people"[12] While not flagging the reference for the ordinary viewer, the first half of the phrase is from an old gospel hymn. Bush often used religious discourse in the public sphere, which delighted many U.S. citizens while offending and frightening others.

On the other extreme is the speech of Ron Reagan, Jr.—the son of the former president—to the Democratic National Convention in 2004, calling for the funding of embryonic stem cell research. According to the analysis of the liberal Protestant magazine *Christian Century*, Reagan said that opponents of stem cell research were "well-meaning and sincere" and are "entitled" to their beliefs about the moral value of embryos, "but it does not follow that the theology of a few should be allowed to forestall the health and well-being of the many. . . . To proceed with research is to be on the side of 'reason,' as opposed to 'ignorance.'" As the *Christian Century* concludes, Reagan "relegates strong moral beliefs to the private sphere—one is 'entitled' to have such beliefs, but to argue for them in public is to force them on 'the many' who don't share them" while labeling claims "he disagrees with a 'theology,' thereby both eliminating the need to argue with it (since presumably it is beyond rational discussion) and insinuating that those who press such a claim are guilty of religious coercion."[13] Despite the complaints of the *Christian Century*, it is a commonly held position that you cannot give religious justifications for your arguments in public debate. What you have here are two approaches, among many, to how religious discourse can be used in the public sphere. To really understand how religious discourse could lead to a lack of conversation, we must look at approaches to religious diversity in the United States.

Religious Diversity and Privatization

Religious diversity means that there are many different religious groups who are in contact with each other, typically within a limited geographic area. The United States is religiously diverse, with 80 percent of Americans who are Christians, 13.5 percent with "no religion," 1.5 percent who are Jewish, eight-tenths of 1 percent who are Buddhist, four-tenths of 1 percent who are Hindu, six-tenths of 1 percent who are Muslim, and 1.6 percent who are "other."[14] Among those 80 percent who are Christians, there are religious liberals and religious conservatives among Catholics and Protestants, as well as subtraditions such as Methodism and Presbyterianism. The United States is, at least compared with many other countries, religiously diverse, and no specific tradition can claim a majority of the citizens.

Historically, the problem with diversity has been, to oversimplify, that people with different religious views may not be able to cooperate. At best they will not be able to have discussions in the public sphere and form a common mind, and at worst they will not be able to stop killing each other. Religions themselves have had different approaches to the problem of religious diversity. One religious solution—"perfectionism"—holds that it is good to live a coherent ethical life, the religious people have a substantive vision of such a life, and they hold that both state and society should help people to achieve this.[15] One way this is done is by limiting the development of competing value spheres: not only other religions but also competing secular ideas. For example, currently in some Muslim countries, perfectionism is enforced by making the practice of competing religions illegal, such as Iran's persecution of people of the Baha'i faith.[16] Similarly, the religiously based wars of the sixteenth and seventeenth centuries in Europe, according to British historian Paul Johnson, "were based on the assumption that only a unitary society was tolerable, and those who did not conform to the prevailing norms, and who could not be forced or terrified into doing so, should be treated as second-class citizens, expelled, or killed."[17]

As opposed to solving the challenges of diversity by avoiding or eliminating diversity, modern secular philosophies "are resigned to the impossibility of integrating the diverse value spheres into a commonly accepted, ethically coherent order."[18] The most influential of these philosophies for the United States is political liberalism, a procedural framework where individuals have the freedom to pursue their own vision of the good, as long as they do not interfere with others. The founders of the United States were deeply steeped in these ideas, and the United States became the epitome of a liberal democratic state. In principle, the government does not try to determine your values, but gives you the freedom to pursue your values as long as you do not interfere with others. Most influential religions in the United States have been either strong supporters of political liberalism or have made some sort of accommodation with liberalism.[19]

In principle, one feature of liberalism is that religion is relegated to the private sphere of the individual, where there is no danger that religion could end up imposing one particular version of the good on others. Religion becomes "personal," a part of an individual's subjective opinion and interests and, most specifically, not a part of debates in the public sphere.

This privatization has grown over time. Structurally, religion had an official role in the public sphere with the established state churches from the colonial era until 1833 when Massachusetts became the last state to end its official establishment. Unofficially, long after the last state establishment fell it was not considered wrong to have strong religious influence in public affairs, as long as it was the "right" type of religious influence. From the colonial period until the 1960s, Protestantism was the "right" type, and Protestants were the unofficial guardians of the public sphere, having de facto control over a number of institutions. Catholics and Jews were marginalized but often tried to influence political life. To take an obvious example of Protestant hegemony, the first non-Protestant president was elected in 1960.

Perhaps even more important, religion has been used to great effect to challenge the state. The struggle to free the slaves in the nineteenth century was motivated largely by religious feelings and argued for with "God talk." If we look at the twentieth-century civil rights movement, we see figures such as the Reverend Martin Luther King using "God talk" to both mobilize followers and justify arguments. However, by the late 1960s, the explicit influence of religion in public life appeared to be in decline. Theorists such as Thomas Luckmann were even predicting that religious privatization would become essentially complete, with religion entirely withdrawing into a privatized subjective space and not influencing any other institution.[20]

The emergence of evangelical Protestants in politics in the late 1970s—displacing the more secular-sounding mainline Protestants—made people wonder whether privatization was really occurring. For example, in his study of public religions around the world, José Casanova concluded that "privatization is not a modern structural trend but, rather, a historical option. To be sure, it seems to be a modern 'preferred option,' but it is an option nonetheless."[21] The United States does not seem to be taking the privatization option, because religious discourse continues in the public sphere.

Evidence also suggests that Americans do not want religion to be totally privatized. For example, in a 2000 survey, 75 percent of the general public said they thought it was okay for political candidates to talk publicly about their religious views, 87 percent favored religious congregations "working with" government agencies for social service provision, 72 percent favored congregations "receiving government funds" to provide services for the poor, 78 percent favored religious congregations making statement to public officials on topics of concern to the community, and 72 percent favored congregations sponsoring meetings to which public officials are invited. For more explicitly using religious discourse to influence public policy, there is a lesser degree of support, but remains quite strong. Respondents were asked if they wanted religious groups to take a more active role in "bringing religious values to bear on public policy": 49 percent said "more active," and 40 percent said "less active."[22] In another survey, participants were asked, "Should religion be a private matter, one that should be kept out of public debate over social and political issues?":

66 percent of the public said it should be kept out, and 34 percent kept in. This masks great variation with 68 percent of churchgoing evangelicals saying religion should be kept *in*, and 85 percent of nonreligious respondents saying it should be kept *out*.[23] This degree of support of and opposition to privatization has been stable over time. The public has repeatedly been asked by pollsters, "Should churches express views on political matters?"; 48 percent said yes in March of 1957, and 51 percent said yes in August 2004.[24]

A good portion of the public clearly believes in using religious discourse in the public sphere. But, will this use lead to lessened conversation? Since I am interested in discussions among citizens in the public sphere, where they would come to a "common mind" about "matters of common interest," I asked the respondents about a conversation with a neighbor with the following question: "So, you are Catholic [or Baptist or whatever their actual religious identity], and you have your particularly Catholic [or Baptist, etc.] way of thinking about these issues. Let's say that your next door neighbor is from India, and they practice the Hindu religion, and they have a Hindu way of thinking about these issues. Let's also say that you are having a conversation with them about genetics. Should you explain your position on these issues using religious terms or secular terms?"[25] From this question, we can determine whether people will bring religion into a debate in a way that stunts communication.[26]

Respondents, by and large, liked the idea of discussing RGTs with the Hindu neighbor. Reflecting the growing diversity of the country, a large portion of the respondents spontaneously gave their own example of a Hindu neighbor, coworker or acquaintance, or a person from another religion they considered to be quite different from theirs. Many displayed a fairly good surface-level knowledge of Hinduism, with some joking that when the Hindu neighbors come over for the barbeque, they won't serve beef.

In rough congruence with the public opinion polls described above, a solid majority of the people with whom we spoke thought you should use religious discourse with the Hindu neighbor. The breakdown by religious tradition mirrors the public opinion surveys as well: most conservative Protestants would use religious discourse with the Hindu neighbor, a majority of Catholics; about half of mainline Protestants and a minority of Jews. A majority of the secular respondents, surprisingly (and I will develop this below), also thought that one should use religious discourse with the neighbor.

What the people we interviewed did *not* say is important. Not a single person said that they should use religious language because they have religious truth, the neighbor does not, and the neighbor needs to be taught the truth. There is no doubt that some of the respondents *think* that they have religious truth and that they should be imparting it to others, but this would be, in my opinion, a small group. (It is notable that if they think this they do not feel it is publicly legitimate to say this to a stranger.) My respondents are similar to those of Alan Wolfe who, in his study, found that the vast majority of middle-class Americans are very much concerned with basic civility. Wolfe found that what bothered his respondents the most "is the idea of excluding others who may not share one's particular religious commitments."[27]

We also encountered no separatists who said they would not talk to someone who was Hindu. Obviously, because we started the recruitment of respondents through congregations, if a congregation's leadership advocated separatism, they would not have given us any of their congregants' names. Therefore, we can at least imagine that some fundamentalist congregations have tendencies toward separatism, but if so, they would not be involved in public discussions anyway. My conclusion is that there are almost no separatists in the American religious traditions that I examined who a priori do not want to talk with people from other religions.

Advocating the Use of Secular Discourse with the Hindu Neighbor

A distinct minority thought that the conversation with the Hindu neighbor should be kept on a secular level. There were two dominant reasons given for this stance. The first was a concern about offending others. This is the embodiment of the classic admonishment to not discuss sex, religion, and politics in polite company—and the topic at hand involves all three. It also mirrors the concerns in the literature of political theory and culture wars. Institutionally, this response most often comes from Catholics and Jews, suggesting that this is actually not so much a statement of not wanting to cause offense by imposing *their* religion on others, but rather a reaction to the Protestant majority historically imposing their religion (and causing offense) to Jews and Catholics.[28] For example, when asked if he should speak "nonreligiously" to the Hindu neighbor, a reconstructionist Jewish nurse said simply, "I get a little turned off when people talk to me [in] a religious way, I guess, so, I'm 'non'."

Those who did not want to give offense or impose saw the primary problem as maintaining your religious beliefs while speaking a secular language. Paul, the fundamentalist man whom we met in earlier chapters, laid out the primary tension:

> Well, I guess you always want to use your religion. I mean you want to have it in your mind, but then you don't want to push it on people 'cause people get upset. And like religion or politics, people—they get mad [at it]. So you don't want to stick it in their faces, but then you don't want to give up your belief. And you have to do it in a way that you're thinking straight. You don't want to tell people what to do. . . . You know, but you don't want to give up your thoughts. But you don't want to act like you're Mr. know-it-all, and you know everything. Because everybody thinks differently. And that's a problem with all these things—because everybody has their own thoughts.

Similarly, a Catholic lawyer said:

> Well, if we were discussing it, I would try and—well, I don't think I can do it in completely secular terms because my position is not one that is secular. I mean I think that I would try and phrase the conversation as religiously neutral as I could because I have no clue what a Hindu would think about these issues. . . . I don't think that it's particularly productive for me to hold out my Catholicity as being somehow—as having some sort of intellectual or moral superiority to his position.

The second major reason given for secular discussion with the neighbor is that, if people used their religious discourses, they would not understand each other. That is, many respondents were concerned with the problem of mutual intelligibility identified by political theorists. However, they were not concerned with a lack of understanding leading to diminished conversation, but rather their concern was pragmatic: respondents assumed they were trying to get the Hindu neighbor to agree with their viewpoint about RGTs, and that if the neighbor did not understand the arguments, the arguments would not work. For example, Keith, a young secular man with whom we spoke, said that he wanted to use "universal facts," which are,

> facts that are understood and could be understood by anybody. When you say that "scripture" says, well a Buddhist does not care, or does not even under-

stand because they have never read the Bible. So it would be difficult to get your point of view across even though it was completely appropriate in this particular person's mind and clear in their mind of what they were trying to say. It would be not understandable by anybody.

Advocating the Use of Religious Discourse with the Hindu Neighbor

As you can see from above, some of the respondents who want to use secular discourse are not sure they can do it. The rest of the respondents do not even want to try. By far the most prevalent reason for advocating the use of religious discourse is that using only secular discourse is not possible. However, while the image we have of the religious antiabortion advocate is that he or she would be speaking explicit theology, scaring off potential discussion partners, the reality is more subtle.

Religious Discourse as Legitimation for Secular Claims

Through the media we are often shown a group of people from the same religion speaking about social issues using explicitly religious discourse. For example, in recent years the public has been shown internal debates within the Episcopal Church over the consecration of a gay bishop. Opponents of his consecration argued that the Bible prohibits homosexuality, whereas proponents of his consecration argued that the Bible does not prohibit homosexuality, but rather requires us to break down social barriers that lead to discrimination. Similarly, in the initial attempts to build an RGT debate in the public sphere, conservative activists use explicitly religious discourse when talking to people of the same religion. For example, the top of the "Sanctity of Human Life Fact Sheet—2004" published by the Southern Baptist Convention starts with explicitly religious discourse—nine biblical quotes that they see as biblical arguments against abortion. Only later does the fact sheet get to decrying "designer babies" produced with preimplantation genetic diagnosis.[29] If this pattern held for public conversations in mixed religious settings, we would expect that if an evangelical Presbyterian, for example, were having a discussion with the Hindu neighbor, the first words over the fence would be the Apostle's Creed, followed by the Nicene Creed, and finally a few Bible quotes.[30] Then the discussion about RGTs would begin.

However, the religious citizens do not want to use explicitly religious discourse as their primary language in mixed company. Theologian Robin Lovin notes that religious discourse in public life is

> usually a language of legitimation, not a language of persuasion. Whether it comes in the form of "good night and God bless you," at the close of a presidential address, or the recollection of the prophets' cry for justice at a protest rally, religious language enters public speech when the speaker has some confidence that the audience already agrees. The speakers may call for stability or change, for freedom, order, or justice, but they will seldom call for it in God's name until they are sure that they have enlisted their hearers' self-interest on other grounds.[31]

Lovin sees religious discourse as a justifying language used after secular arguments have made the case. However, while Lovin sees religious discourse as used to legitimate claims *after* agreement has been reached, among those with whom we spoke, religious discourse is a means to legitimate secular claims when the claims are not accepted or understood.

Therefore, the majority of the respondents who wanted to use religious discourse in their conversation with the Hindu neighbor did not want to start with religion, but wanted to start talking on a secular level, with what they thought of as shared discursive ground that liberal theorists would suggest. The difference between these respondents and those who wanted to keep religion out of the discussion is that these respondents thought that it would be impossible to keep religion out if the conversation progressed. They would start with saying, for example, "Well, I really think people should avoid having children with cystic fibrosis." If pressed, they would say, "Because it is terrible for children to suffer like that." If pressed as to why we should avoid suffering, if, in other words, forced to legitimate their claim, they would fall back on their religious discourse and say, "In my religious tradition, we are called upon by God to heal the suffering of the world." If asked to further explain, eventually they would get to something more theologically abstract, like the ideas expressed in the Nicene Creed.

Most thought that there would be moments in the conversation with the Hindu neighbor where secular discourse would no longer work. For example, a middle-aged evangelical man said that he tries to avoid "Christian speak" because "nobody knows what the heck you are talking about. It sounds weird. But at the same time too, I would not avoid discussing this because I sort of see my faith and views with the rest of my life, I mean, it's going to come up. . . . But I would hopefully use language they will understand."

Similarly, Wayne is a traditional evangelical who attends church about three times a month, and he is opposed to almost all the RGTs we discussed. When asked the Hindu neighbor question, he first joked that "he has a friend from India, and that this person "definitely has a different mind set." He continued that

> I wouldn't be afraid to discuss the religious aspects of it because I think we're really coming from a totally different religious bases also, and not just culturally. The reason I believe what I believe is that I do believe in the God of the Bible and he believes in a thousand gods and his whole idea of the soul or whatever is totally different from mine. So there would have to be a lot of discussion that went into it.

So far, Wayne sounds like he is going to start the conversation with religious discourse, but he continues that

> there are certain practical issues or questions that I suppose I could bring out to make him think about it. But somewhere along the way, the reason I believe what I believe would have to come out, probably in order to really convey my thoughts on that. I believe that there is a God who created man, who created nature, and has an intent for us, has a life for us, provided a salvation for us, and cares about us as opposed to a thousand gods that are warring with each other. . . . Just a whole different perspective on things. So yes, I think I would have to bring that out at some point.

The key is that you "would have to bring that out *at some point.*" It is inevitable, says Wayne, that as we move from "practical issues or questions," he would have to refer to his religious beliefs so that "he can really convey my thoughts on that."

Lisa attends a nontraditional evangelical megachurch, the kind that performs plays instead of giving sermons and provides Starbucks coffee during the service. She is very active in the congregation, attending every Sunday, and having taught Sunday school for many years and leading Bible studies. Like most evangelicals, religion was front and center to her thinking about many issues. When we asked her whether people should use a nonreligious way of talking to others in public as we debate these technologies, she said:

Wisdom would dictate that they not use strictly religious terms because that's alienating and it smacks of superiority and exclusivity and all those things and I think that's unwise. I think it's perfectly fine to say "this is what I believe because this is really what I believe and it's based upon God's way. I really believe he's there and really believe he has opinions and has revealed those things in his word." But then also to say "but I also believe that common sense would dictate that" and on and on. Or "our experience would show that, you know, that we don't want to create a perfect race" or you know, whatever. . . . You know, someone would get up there and pound, you know, thump Jesus down this road and that's offensive. That's offensive to me and I believe in him. So I think we need to be careful when we're talking about these things.

Bruce, a self-identified liberal Catholic, has similar views. He would start the conversation, but would ultimately have to turn to his religious reasons. He said, "The only thing that I can address is what I live, you know, that's all I can speak to and if I have a reason for thinking something is wrong, then, if they want to hear it, I'll share it with them. . . . I mean I can't just say it's wrong and not have a reason for it. . . . But, you know, if I felt strongly about something and you wanted to hear why, then, I would give you a reason otherwise I wouldn't have a strong opinion."

The Inability to Separate

These people also said that you had to use religious discourse because this is what you truly believed. Many respondents had the briefest of statements about this, suggesting it was obvious to them. For example, we spoke with a Pentecostal woman who said that she would use religious discourse because "that's who I am . . . so that's probably how it would come across." Sheryl, a traditional evangelical who attended services weekly, went into more detail. She was supportive of most RGTs. She paused for a few seconds in thought after being presented with the Hindu neighbor scenario and then said that it is inevitable that she uses her religious discourse:

I usually tell people "my value system is this so you need to know that's where I'm coming from." So I'm consistent with and if I'm not then people let me know. It's a good thing. . . . I can't separate that because my spiritual beliefs influence everything I do and say. If I really feel that that's the core of who I am, then to say "it only influences me some of the time" is a mistake. So if they are

my neighbors, they would know that anyway. . . . I don't like "preachy." In fact,
I don't get "preachy."

Like the others, she clearly thinks of her religious discourse as something
she would need to use for legitimation.

Michele, a stay-at-home mom with three kids, considers herself to be
a traditionalist Catholic. She also saw no other way to explain herself in
public. Like most of the respondents who wanted to use religious discourse, she cannot help speaking religiously and wants to be tolerant and
accepting of people with other religions. She, like the others, said she has
no choice but to use religious discourse because "that's how I look at it."
But, she continued, "I would respect the fact that they have their religious
beliefs, which come into play. We went to a wedding about a year ago that
was an Afghani couple and—I mean, they believe in God but He has a
different name in their language, you know, we respect that. I mean we
don't agree with their religious beliefs personally, but it doesn't mean that
we disrespect them for that."

Michele's concern with being "respectful"—related to Sheryl's concern
with not being "preachy" is prevalent among people who say they must
speak religiously. They cannot divorce who they are, but want to make
sure that others' religious views are respected. Again, as noted above,
their motivation for using religion was to be able to fully explain or justify
their secularly stated positions, instead of a desire to directly propagate
the faith.

The Curious Case of the Nonreligious

Conservative Protestants, Catholics, and (surprisingly) the secular respondents were more likely to claim that it was acceptable for people to use
religious discourse than were Mainline Protestants and Jews. The pattern
within the religious traditions is consistent with their previous practices.
Mainline Protestantism has been a defender of the liberal democratic
public sphere, promoting liberal values such as "individualism, freedom,
pluralism, tolerance, democracy and intellectual inquiry" in the broader
culture.[32] Mainline Protestantism has also, at least for the past half century,
been acutely sensitive to not "pushing" their views on others—they aspire
to be "the quiet hand of God."[33] RGTs are another situation, analogous
to many previous cases where mainliners have not wanted to push their
views on others. Mainline Protestant theology is also more privatized, in

that mainliners can more easily treat the religion as something they do on Sundays but does not influence every aspect of their lives. Jews, as a religious minority, have probably always been privatized in the United States, in that attempts at speaking Jewish discourse in the public sphere would either be ignored or possibly be dangerous.

It is harder to understand why the nonreligious respondents were just as likely to think one should use religious discourse with the Hindu neighbor as were conservative Protestants and Catholics. Examining their responses, it is clear that like conservative Protestants and Catholics, the nonreligious agree that a religious view and a secular view cannot be detangled. However, unlike these groups, the nonreligious respondents seem primarily concerned with fairness.

I actually changed the question slightly for the nonreligious respondents because it was implausible that *they* would want to speak religious discourse to the person next door with the different religion. Instead, I asked them about the case where the neighbor was making a religious argument to *them*. I also changed that person from being a Hindu to being a "devout Catholic" to try to make the neighbor in a position of discursive power and make the nonreligious respondent the one who is potentially put upon—an attempt to match the power differential between the Christian and the Hindu in the scenario given to the Christian respondents. This difference in question wording should bias the results even more toward the nonreligious respondents wanting to keep religion out of the public sphere, because in their scenario, they are the ones who are being oppressed.

But, like their religious counterparts, they also did not see how the devout Catholic neighbor could separate their views. Matthew, who approved of almost all RGTs, said that it "would be okay if they used religious arguments because that's one of the foundations of how they see things. It's how they make their arguments so that would be fine." Karina, a young woman who works in health care, emphasized that this is not how she sees the world, but "their religious points are their belief systems so I think it would be okay. . . . That's what their values are based on so I think it'd be okay for them to use that as an argument of theirs, or back up an argument of theirs."

Sadie, a teacher, told me that the neighbor *cannot* use secular discourse because religion is "the basis for the formation of their ideas." Sadie then told me about her friend Louise, who is Catholic.

We agree on nothing. It's absolutely hysterical. So, would I expect her to eliminate that? Never. That's what makes her her. That's where she has her opinions.

I can't ask her to step out of the church. . . . But I certainly respect her and I can't imagine having a conversation with anyone that doesn't bring their whole life to the table. You can't amputate parts of your life to have a good discussion. It wouldn't be a good discussion if you didn't bring that into it.

Most of the nonreligious respondents would finish by saying something like "but the devout Catholic is not going to convince me that they are right." Yet, they want them to have the chance to try, using their own language. That is, the nonreligious respondents seem to be in favor of religious discourse in politics out a sense of fairness, which itself seems to have developed from having their nonreligious views looked down on in public debates.[34]

For example, Ruth, a young woman who works in social service provision says, "I would expect them to use religious arguments if they are a devout Catholic because religion plays a large part, or nonreligion plays a large part, in our values and beliefs. . . . But I would hope that just as I think it's okay that they impart their religion, they would respect my non-imparting of religion." Another nonreligious respondent said, "Of course it would be okay if they made religious arguments about this. They have a right to express their opinion. I probably won't agree with it and will counter, but they have every right to express their opinion." Another said that the neighbor "should use her religious arguments, absolutely." When asked why, she replied: "Well, why not? If she is devout and if religion is a significant part of her life and that religion forms her opinions, then I should be the first person to say, 'bring them on. Let me hear them.' I think that's not only great spirit, but I think that's fairness." Another said that they "can use anything they want . . . I'm a pretty big believer in freedom of speech. . . . I think you can use any argument you want, whether or not it will be a persuasive one is another matter."

Inverting the Intelligibility Argument

Religious discourse is used by religious people to both legitimate their secular claims and to make themselves better understood, since they cannot create separate religious and secular selves. Note that using religious discourse to make yourself better understood is an inversion of the view of political theorists that religious discourse must be excluded from arguments so that we can understand each other and have an effective discussion. Instead, respondents seem to believe that since RGTs have religious implications, and because they do not think you can wall off your religious self from your public discourse, to try to explain your position without religion is insincere, and insincerity diminishes understanding.

Perhaps it should not surprise us that Americans think that this is important. As anthropologist Joel Robbins has argued, a "sincerity culture" is one of the linguistic features of modernity. Indeed, this rise in the importance of sincerity in communication—in place of earlier notions of honor and courtesy—first occurred as a side effect of the Protestant Reformation. Robbins writes, "Expressing the truth about one's inner states in everyday conversation and conduct became a value in a way that it had not been before. . . . Protestantism would develop this emerging cult of sincerity to an impressive extent, taking a nascent version of . . . a 'sincerity culture' and making it a cornerstone of modern views of the self, of social life, and . . . language."[35] If this notion did originate in Protestantism—and its historical origins are not important to us here—it has spread to be a general belief held by the citizens in the modern United States.

To see the importance of this sincerity in argumentation to the religious community in the United States, consider Rudy, a middle-aged man who identifies himself as a traditionalist Catholic. He says that he would want to have a religious conversation with the neighbor "because I think it's important that people know why you are that way. Why do you think in those terms? I think it's important that I'm not bragging I'm Catholic but I'm not ashamed either. It's just who I am. So I think I would want them to know that." Andrew, a middle-aged white traditional evangelical who is in sales, is concerned about being "disingenuous." Andrew said, "It would be disingenuous to use strictly secular terms. I wouldn't want them to explain their decision to me without their faith being part of it so I think we both ought to be able to use faith terms to understand the decision making." Similarly, Susan, a mainline Protestant nurse, said, "I think you should share what your faith brings to this decision or this problem. I don't know much about the Hindu faith. But I think we should not be bashful about sharing our faith, how it influences us and why."

Will Religious Discourse Lead to a Lack of Debate?

This book has examined how an RGT debate may not occur because of the inability or unwillingness of people to deliberate due to a lack of shared discourses. Religious discourse has long been thought of as the least shared discourse. Political theorists have long advocated various degrees of removal of religion from the public sphere partially due to concerns of an inability to communicate, evolving into more serious balkanization of society. Similarly, culture wars theories presume that referring to religious discourse will make people want to stop talking because exposure to other religious worldviews threatens their own.

Examination of the interviews shows, first, that people want to talk with people from other religious traditions about RGTs, as well as about the religious presuppositions behind their views about RGTs. Even the respondents from the most separatist religious tradition in the sample— Protestant fundamentalism—do not mind talking with people with entirely different religious perspectives. There is also a strong commitment to this very American idea that "you can say anything you want to me, I just don't have to be convinced by you." Respondents, even secular respondents, are very concerned that religious people be given a fair chance to tell their religious views to everyone.

Part of the religious population does not want to use religious discourse at all, and the other part wants to start with secular claims and then only use religious claims if needed for justification. Therefore, the involvement of religious people in an RGT debate will not have as much religious discourse in it as we might think. It would only be during an in-depth conversation that religion would ultimately emerge.

But, even this lesser amount of religious discourse does not seem to have the problems theorists associate with it. Respondents seem to see exposure to religious discourse as inevitably part of deliberation in the United States, because they think that religious beliefs cannot be separated from secular beliefs. Moreover, they do not view religion as impeding mutual understanding, but contributing to it if the speaker is indeed religious. When they themselves speak religiously, it would be to make sure that the conversation partner understands their otherwise secular claims. Even secular people with whom we spoke say that if someone is religious, then they should speak religiously, so that everyone can truly understand their claims. To do otherwise is insincere. Religious discourse would then at least be neutral in facilitating deliberation and thus the formation of the collective mind in the public sphere. If deliberation about RGTs is limited in the public sphere, it does not appear that it will be the result of the religious nature of the discourse used.

There is no question that many people do not want to hear religious discourse in the public sphere and that religious minorities find it alienating. That may be a reason, on justice grounds alone, to not allow religious discourse in the public sphere, but that concern does not speak to my concerns about a diminished public debate. Moreover, I want to limit the conclusion about religious discourse in the public sphere to a debate about RGTs. There may well be other issues, perhaps that are more clearly connected to religion in the public mind, where religious discourse would have the negative effects described by theorists. For example, there is no denying that there has been religiously motivated violence in public, such as riots in the nineteenth century between Catholics and Protestants over Bible reading in schools. But, for our purposes, concerns that people will not want to discuss RGTs because of the use of religious discourse seem overblown.

CHAPTER EIGHT

Conclusions

It seems that every day we hear of a new technological achievement in human reproduction. These emerge at a dizzying speed, with very little or no opportunity for the public to debate their merits. Indeed, the issues under examination in this book may soon seem very tame and taken for granted, with even more spectacular technological possibilities becoming the new topics of debate. For example, scientists in Britain are creating hybrid human-cow embryos for research, and work continues on artificial wombs.[1] However, there will be a debate in the future about reproductive genetic technologies (RGTs), which will involve the religious citizens.

How RGTs Are Opposed

If we look across all the religious respondents with whom we spoke, we see a range of discourses frequently used to oppose RGTs. The first and probably most anticipated is the embryonic life discourse. Since many of the RGTs result in embryonic death, it is not surprising that many people use the embryonic life discourse to oppose the use of these RGTs. In my more technical terms, many respondents consider RGTs like preimplantation genetic diagnosis to be analogous to abortion for cystic fibrosis, so they use the same discourse they use to oppose abortion.

I did not as clearly anticipate finding the extensive use of discourses about nature, God, and humanity. There are a number of nature discourses that people use to oppose RGTs, such as what I call "secular nature," a general preference for following what is perceived as "natural." Other respondents use a natural law discourse, where they oppose RGTs that result in changes from the way human beings are naturally supposed to be. In the hubris discourse, there is no task that is inherently left to God, and humans are supposed to improve their situation, but the key is to figure out which human changes God would like. While these are discourses used to oppose RGTs, the discourse used by those opposed to the most RGTs is the Promethean fatalist discourse, where humans are not to usurp God's plans for us. This Promethean fatalist discourse is not used for everything that God created, such as, presumably, deadly diseases, but in contrast to how it is used in public bioethical debate, healing disease is one of the tasks God leaves to humans. Enhancements are treading into God's area of authority.

Discourses of human dignity and equality of treatment also were often used to oppose RGTs. In the social dignity/inequality discourse, social groups such as class or sex are under consideration when evaluating equality, which is used by the (relative) supporters to oppose enhancements. The individual dignity/equality discourse is used by those most opposed to RGTs, and picking between any two individuals, unrelated to the groups they are in, is what is problematic.

That suffering has no purpose and needs to be eradicated is the most pervasive and deeply assumed discourse among proponents of RGTs. This is also a discourse that almost everybody seems to use at some point, if only to describe a reaction to the flu. However, this discourse has a competitor taught in the Christian tradition where suffering has meaning and therefore should not necessarily be eradicated. I found in chapter 6 that the discourse of meaningful suffering is used by the strongest opponents of RGTs, where suffering can be pedagogical for either the sufferer or those around the sufferer. The use of this discourse by the religious—particularly religious conservatives—partially explains why these citizens are opposed to a broader range of RGT applications than are nonreligious persons. While not in favor of all suffering, and thus at least sometimes using the medical discourse of suffering, people who use the meaningful suffering discourse are more likely to think of borderline cases such as early-onset Alzheimer's disease or obesity as producing meaningful suffering and then oppose applications of RGTs that would alleviate these conditions. In everyday terms, these four discourses are the reasons why religious people are disproportionately opposed to RGTs.

The Mystery of Human Genetic Engineering for Cystic Fibrosis

The particular technology of human genetic engineering for cystic fibrosis did not follow my initial expectations. For the non–pro-lifers who are also the (relative) proponents of RGTs, human genetic engineering for cystic fibrosis is in the health domain with other RGTs that relieve what is considered to be serious disease. They then use the same medical discourse of suffering to discuss it as they do other "health-related" RGTs, which I expected. Among the people who were opposed to most RGTs, I was surprised to find that they talked about human genetic engineering for cystic fibrosis differently than the other RGTs, often supporting it, while talking of relieving suffering and thus placing it in a distinct domain. Since it is in a distinct domain, which uses a different discourse, it will not be considered part of the abortion or genetic control issue domains and is likely to be considered a separate issue altogether in the public sphere.

Among theologians and religious elites who oppose most RGTs, the conclusions about this one particular application are mixed. For Catholic leaders, it would be acceptable in principle if it could be done without harming embryos or without engaging in any illicit practices like fertilizing embryos outside a woman's body.[2] One possibility would be a shot given to the adults who would then reproduce. Among conservative Protestants, there is no consensus, but some prominent activists are opposed. For example, evangelical anti-RGT activist Nigel M. De S. Cameron and his coauthor use the Promethean fatalist and individual dignity/equality discourses to oppose both enhancement and health applications of human genetic engineering. While God gave dominion over "the rest of creation" to humans, they write, "dominion over humanity still properly belongs to God alone," and human genetic engineering results in humans having dominion over each other. It is a "threat to seize the place of God the creator in designing and redesigning human nature itself," they write.[3] There are also, "as followers of Jesus Christ, . . . practical ethical callings that must frame our consideration of germline interventions" which include that "we are to care for those who are in need, including those who have genetic structures we would consider to be defects." We should be "caring for the least among us, caring for the poor, and loving one another." They continue that we must care for persons with genetic disease, "doing what we are able to do to serve them in their need, and not to decide who needs to be 'fixed' in order to be considered worth living."[4]

Cameron uses many of the strongly oppositional discourses described in this book to oppose human genetic engineering for cystic fibrosis, but why don't the ordinary respondents use these discourses, particularly the evangelicals who share a tradition with Cameron and who disproportionately reside on the left side of figure 3? The key question is as follows: Why would preimplantation genetic diagnosis for cystic fibrosis be described using the three most oppositional discourses such as Promethean fatalism ("it is usurping God's role") while human genetic engineering for cystic fibrosis is like "a vaccination?"

One possible answer is that human genetic engineering for cystic fibrosis was the only RGT health application for a severe disease we asked about that did not involve destroying embryos, and this feature may be the salient difference from preimplantation genetic diagnosis. In other words, it could be that it takes a very strong nonnegotiable discourse like embryonic life to counteract the power of the medical discourse of suffering in contemporary U.S. society. If that is the case, then what is more mysterious is why the other three discourses, which were often used for enhancements when embryos were not at risk, could not be used by themselves to argue against "health."

Another possibility is that it is not embryonic life that creates the distinction between the two technologies for avoiding cystic fibrosis, but that human genetic engineering was the only technology portrayed as a modification of an existing person to improve health, instead of choosing to bring a healthier person into existence (preimplantation genetic diagnosis). (People who use the embryonic life discourse would say that modified embryos are existing persons.) If this is the case, then the use of the discourses is more constrained than I had been portraying, in that they apparently are not used for situations involving the health of existing human bodies. Promethean fatalism does not fit with healing bodies as God has already given us dominion over medical care; individual dignity/equality is not about "picking and choosing" between health conditions in existing bodies; and the suffering caused by disease in existing bodies is not meaningful. While I cannot offer definitive proof that it is the existing persons versus bringing into existence distinction that matters between preimplantation genetic diagnosis and human genetic engineering for cystic fibrosis, there is a good deal of evidence for this interpretation.

First, consider the smaller non–pro-lifer group that I separately analyzed in chapters 4–6. They are typically opposed to almost all RGTs, but
never say that life begins at conception. For this group, the distinction
between preimplantation genetic diagnosis and human genetic engineering for cystic fibrosis is not about embryonic death, but something else,
because these people are not concerned with embryonic death per se and
they still make the distinction between these two applications.

Second, when discussing human genetic engineering for cystic fibrosis, respondents made analogies to modifying an existing person to make
her or her offspring more healthy. The primary previous situation that
people made analogies to is vaccinations, such as polio and smallpox,
where something was done to an existing person by a doctor so that other
people would be healthy. People also made analogies to surgeries and
pharmaceuticals, which are also medical treatments for existing persons.

Third, this interpretation parallels a long-standing distinction in bioethical debate, with the conservative bioethicists—who would fit best with
the pro-lifers on the left side of figure 3—making the same distinctions.
In bioethics, the traditional moral line between health and enhancement
is at restoring "normal human functioning." There used to be a consensus that enhancement was any genetic change that would result in traits
that any human does not currently possess. This would allow for changing
disease causing genes because most humans have normal copies of those
genes, but would not allow for superintelligence or superstrength that no
human possesses.

The normal functioning concept assumes that we can start with the
existing body to decide what is ethical, but people in the human genetic
engineering debate have begun to move away from this by looking to the
medical profession to define what is and is not a disease. The impetus for
this move is that human genetic engineering applications such as making people genetically less susceptible to cancer is not a "species-typical
function," but has long been a goal of medicine.[5] Therefore, the therapy/
enhancement divide is coming to be redefined from "normal functioning"
to avoiding any condition that the medical profession defines as a disease,
regardless of current bodies.

On the other hand, conservative and religious bioethicists have tried
to reground the "normal," and thus medical care, in the existing human
body. For example, Francis Fukuyama considers enhancement to be creating a posthuman species and wants to limit genetic technology to promoting health. His ideas of what is "typical of the human species" are

complex, but he is trying to fix the enhancement/therapy distinction in its old location of what is currently possible, given the existing genes in the human species. He then argues for "therapeutic" or health uses and excludes "enhancement" as resulting in the posthuman society.[6] Because religious and conservative bioethicists are trying to constrain medicine to modifying existing bodies, it is not surprising that the same impulse exists among ordinary religious conservatives.

If I am right, then human genetic engineering for cystic fibrosis is in a different issue domain—and the discourses used for the other RGTs are not used for it—because it is the only health-promoting RGT that treats existing "bodies." The offshoot of this subtle distinction is that if a scientist figures out how to make healthier people come into existence, even if there is no embryonic death, religious people would oppose this technology using one of the three discourses. But, producing the same result through genetically changing existing people—which strikes people as "medicine"—would be acceptable.

The Meaning of "Health" in Other Studies of the Public's Views of RGTs

Therefore, other studies of the public's views of RGTs may need to define "health" more precisely. These other studies provide many difficult to weave together descriptions of the structure of public opinion about RGTs, but one generalization is consistent across studies—the public generally accepts what they define as "health" applications of RGTs and opposes "enhancement" RGTs. Of course, everyone draws this line in a different place, but they mostly have this morally significant line. This is akin to saying that people have two issue domains: health and enhancement, and they have different conclusions (and discourses) in each domain.

The data presented in the previous chapters would suggest something similar for the religious respondents. Everyone had a distinct "health" issue domain where they approved of the technology and an opposition to genetic control or opposition to genetic enhancement issue domain where they did not (fig. 3). For the pro-lifers, typically all but human genetic engineering for cystic fibrosis was in the opposition to genetic control domain where the four strongly oppositional discourses were used. For a small subset of the non–pro-lifers, they had the same "opposition to genetic control" domain as the pro-lifers, and the larger group had only enhancements in the opposed to genetic enhancement domain and all other RGTs in the health domain.

In figure 3, I give these health domains slightly different names to indicate their slightly different meanings. The "health promotion" issue domain is what the other scholars who study society at large have identified. Abortion for cystic fibrosis, preimplantation genetic diagnosis for deafness, and human genetic engineering for cystic fibrosis are all for one group of persons acceptable because they improve the health of someone, be it through bringing a healthier person into the world or modifying an existing person to make them and their offspring healthier. The larger group of the non–pro-lifers use this domain, and this finding fits well with the conclusions of the other studies.

On the other hand, the pro-lifers do not place the same issues in their health-related domain. They oppose abortion and preimplantation genetic diagnosis for cystic fibrosis, but they do approve of human genetic engineering for cystic fibrosis. Their "health" domain is better described as "medicine" and is limited to RGTs where currently existing people are modified to help the health of themselves and their offspring. Therefore, I reach a slightly different conclusion about the health/enhancement distinction than the other studies.

Understanding the Repugnance toward Reproductive Cloning

Reproductive cloning is in some ways the ultimate RGT because in principle it allows for perfect genetic control by copying an existing person. It is also one of the few technologies that has been banned by some countries, although it is not banned in the United States. It has been the subject of countless ethical writings and therefore deserves some separate commentary.

The cloning of Dolly the sheep in 1997 lead to near-universal condemnation of human reproductive cloning among the public. The public is by far the most familiar with this issue than they are about any of the other technologies that I mentioned, with the exception of amniocentesis for cystic fibrosis followed by abortion. They are also almost uniformly opposed. In the survey, about 89 percent of the public disapproves or strongly disapproves of reproductive cloning, with 99 percent of fundamentalists, 97 percent of evangelicals and 96 percent of both mainliners and traditionalist Catholics being so opposed (see table 2). Each of the discourses under close examination in chapters 4–6 of this book is used to oppose reproductive cloning except embryonic life. (As with human genetic engineering,

we portrayed cloning as not resulting in the death of embryos.)[7] Which-
ever discourse people used to oppose human genetic engineering enhancements were typically used to oppose reproductive cloning.

But, the response was different than that of the responses to the other
RGTs. Leon Kass has famously written about "the wisdom of repugnance" regarding cloning, saying, "Repugnance is the emotional expres-
sion of deep wisdom, beyond reason's power fully to articulate it."[8] The
people with whom we spoke also experience something like repugnance at
the thought of cloning. Is it possible to articulate this sense of repugnance
that Kass ascribes to deep wisdom?

The bioethical debate about cloning offers a number of such reasons
why cloning should not be allowed. First and foremost, cloning would not
be safe at present for the cloned child, especially given the high rate of
malformations in the animals that have been cloned. Another concern is
that the children could be psychologically harmed because of a diminished
sense of individuality. Perhaps people have a right to their own genetic
identity, or to not knowing how their particular genome will "turn out" in
the end. Another concern is that clones would be treated as objects and
not as persons.[9]

I saw little evidence that the public shared the concerns identified by
the professional ethicists. A few people mentioned safety, with the most
informed persons noting that Dolly the cloned sheep had died an earlier
than expected death. The distinguishing feature of cloning, compared to
the other RGTs, is that an exact copy of a person is made, but very few
people dwelled on this characteristic, even though it is a central theme in
media discussions of clones.

"Repugnance" suggests that people find cloning more problematic—
that it strongly violates some deeply held beliefs. I also did not see that
among the interviewees. The utter and rapid dismissal of reproductive
cloning as a legitimate practice was not because cloning was considered to
be a strong violation of beliefs compared to other RGTs, but rather a lack
of an analogy to a situation that would result in supporting cloning.

The difference in response between cloning and the other RGTs was
that there was no weighing, no debating, and no "hmmmm" or pauses in
the conversations. They just said no, or even more strongly would state
that cloning was ridiculous or absurd and then would briefly allude to previous discourses of opposition they had used. Put differently, with cloning
there is no positive argument to weigh against that people wanted to pause
and consider. People are familiar with the situation of protecting your

children from disease, which people find analogous to health applications of RGTs. People are familiar with the situations of "improving" your child's chances in life through making them more "intelligent" by making them study harder or take piano lessons. These later situations are analogous for those who approve of enhancements, and those who disapprove of enhancements are at least aware of those situations and perhaps think of them before rejecting them as proper analogies. But, reproductive cloning does not even evoke either of these previous situations. It is not for health, or even for enhancement. As a woman who attended a nontraditional evangelical church explained, "I guess I just ask the question, 'Why?' Can you imagine the answer that they [the parents] would give you that would make you say, 'Okay, sure.' I couldn't." With no positive "good reason" to engage in reproductive cloning, the discourses that lead to opposition have no competition, and at minimum people's desire for "natural" reproduction wins.

That people lack a reason *for* reproductive cloning, instead of an argument *against*, shows a disjuncture between the public and bioethical debate. We are led by these bioethical debates to think that the near-universal opposition to reproductive cloning must mean that cloning is a particularly glaring case of intervening in God's realm, or will lead to particularly severe affronts to dignity and equality. This is because bioethical arguments start from different premises than the public. The bioethics argument does not start, like the public's, with the assumption that "natural is better." Rather, bioethics debates start with the liberty of scientists to do what they see fit and people to control their bodies as they see fit. In bioethics debates, these premises of liberty can be overridden to impose controls, given good enough reasons, but, opposite to the public's orientation, bioethics has a default position of freedom. We could say that the public says that a new technology is guilty until proven innocent. Professional ethicists say that a new technology is innocent until proven guilty.

In sum, the religious public did not feel the need to justify their conclusions by coming up with reasons why cloning should *not* be allowed. It was up to the proponents to give them a good reason, an analogy with a previous experience that would justify cloning, and they had not heard a good reason from me, or from anywhere else. The religious public is therefore not uniformly opposed to reproductive cloning because it is such a particularly distinct form of RGT, but rather because it is a form of RGT for which there is no obvious positive argument.

Clones as Objects or Products

A much publicized concern with cloning is that we as a society would think of a cloned child as an object or product, somehow less human than us, leading to disastrous results. In theologian Gilbert Meilaender's words, "Once a child becomes a project or product temptations such as using cloned children for their organs will make sense."[10] In Jean Bethke Elshtain's "nightmare scenario" about cloning, she envisions a society which "clones human beings to serve as spare parts. Because the cloned entities are not fully human, our moral queasiness could be disarmed and we could 'harvest' organs to our heart's content."[11] Denominations and theologians worry about this scenario and try to teach that a clone should have the same moral status as everyone else.[12]

We asked a follow-up question to the question about cloning, that is, whether the respondent thought the cloned child would be "just as human as everyone else." Worries about clones being considered less than human seem to be misplaced—the vast majority of people, of whom almost all were opposed to cloning, said that a clone would be just as human as anyone else.[13]

In fact, it seems to be a deeply taken for granted, unquestioned idea, suggesting that it would take a great deal of effort for the public to be convinced otherwise. A classic way of showing students a deeply assumed idea is to ask them to "breach" the normal activities that occur in a situation and see what happens. For example, students are told to act like a stranger in their own home, to attempt to bargain for prices in a grocery store, or to stand six inches away from people in otherwise empty elevators. Strong, incredulous reactions ensue, indicating that they have violated some deep assumption about how society is supposed to work.[14] My question about the humanity of a clone did not evoke the same reaction as standing six inches from someone in an elevator, but people reacted emphatically nonetheless, suggesting that it was deeply assumed that clones would be fully human.

For example, Jim, a self-described moderate Catholic, stated his opposition to cloning. When we followed by asking "Would you consider this cloned child to be just as human as everybody else?" he replied:

JIM: Sure, absolutely.
INTERVIEWER: Why is that?
JIM: Why is that?

INTERVIEWER: Yes. Some people might say, might disagree, and say that they are not human. What would you say to this person?

JIM: Oh God, [what would I say] to the person who says they are not human?

INTERVIEWER: Yes.

JIM: Then how are you going to treat them? Okay, tell me how you are going to treat that person. You're going to treat them inhumane? "Well hell no." "Then shut up." "Then treat them human." "They are human then, aren't they?" "Well I guess they are." "Of course, they are."

The interviewees with whom we spoke usually were not as emphatic as Jim, but just incredulous at the question. Frank, a fundamentalist, responded to the question by saying, "Sure, why not? I can't think of why this child wouldn't be." Similarly, one of the secular respondents was asked the following:

INTERVIEWER: So would you consider a cloned child to be just as human as everyone else?

RESPONDENT: Sure.

INTERVIEWER: Why?

RESPONDENT: It's made just like everybody [else]. I mean, it's made of the same stuff as everybody else.

INTERVIEWER: Someone might disagree and say that they're not human. What would you say to that person?

RESPONDENT: I'd say I don't understand how they cannot be human. It's almost like saying a cake made at home is not a cake. The same ingredients go into it as go into a cake at a restaurant. It's all the same stuff. It's just somebody else putting it in there.

Justine, a secular woman in her mid-fifties said, like the others, that she would consider a cloned child to be just as human as everyone else. She was then asked, "Why? What if someone said that they aren't as human as everyone else because they weren't created through a sex act, that it's not natural?" She retorted, "I would say that you just created another 'ism.' 'A clone is something else to hate' is probably what I'd say to that person who would say that they aren't human."

I do not want to be too Pollyanna-ish here. It is possible that the dehumanization of clones would be a slow and subtle process. Over time, these children could come to be thought of as different from other children, and therefore more likely to be treated as objects and have, for example, their organs removed to given to more fully human children. However, given how the respondents currently talk about cloned children, this process would require much time and effort from someone, and I cannot imagine who would have an interest in teaching people to describe clones as less than human.

Reflexivity and Future Developments

The applicability of the findings in this book for a future RGT debate depends on how this research was designed and implemented, and what unfolds in the future. As for research design, there is not an objective social world that can be directly measured by the analyst, but rather the social world can only be described through the analyst's methods. For example, the findings in all interview-based social science projects are partially determined by the way the questions are asked.

Clearly, given my theoretical model where people use discourses from previous situations that they consider to be analogous, how I describe the technologies in the interview is critical. The future applicability of the findings in this book then depends on these technologies being described in the same way to the public when a broader public debate emerges. All the RGTs, except cloning and human genetic engineering, are currently in use for at least some genetic conditions, so the basic description of the technology is probably going to remain unchanged in the near future. Moreover, the descriptions I choose for the interviews are from the activist and the academic debates, and it is they who will be bringing the debate into the public sphere. The one possible exception is human genetic engineering, which has not been applied to humans, and the details of the technology remain unclear.[15] I have described it like bioethicists have been describing it, but they cannot exactly predict how human genetic engineering will work once it is developed. So, my findings about human genetic engineering will be most accurate in the future to the extent that my description remains correct.

Of course, activists are going to try to teach people to use particular discourses with particular situations of RGTs. Scholars of social movements call this "framing" the debate. For example, in an unrelated public debate, scientists have been trying to teach the public to use the label "somatic cell nuclear transfer" for the process they used to call "therapeutic cloning." In the theoretical terminology of this book, they are trying to move "therapeutic cloning" away from the "genetic control" and "genetic enhancement" domains and into the "health care" domains through avoiding the word "cloning." Similarly, supporters of RGTs will try to make analogies between, for example, preimplantation genetic diagnosis for cystic fibrosis and the medical suffering discourse. This book is then a description of the domains used by people before much of this framing activity has been undertaken.[16]

Will There Be an Effective RGT Debate?

Academic analysis would predict that for pro-lifers the abortion and RGT issues will merge, which would result in the perception by the non–pro-lifers that deliberation about RGTs is pointless because there will be no shared language on which to base a discussion. In the previous chapters, I have shown that such a merger of issues already seems to have happened, not so much through the efforts of activists, but because of how the two issues are described, which results in their being considered to be similar enough to use the same discourses.

However, while I do show that many of the non–pro-lifers do indeed use a separate set of discourses than the pro-lifers to discuss RGTs, there is a large group of the non–pro-lifers who use the same language. This suggests that while many people will feel that starting a conversation is worthless—like the culture war theories would predict—many actually have a discursive basis on which to have that conversation. While James Hunter used his theoretical tradition to predict a total lack of debate (inevitably leading to conflict), I have used a different theoretical tradition and data to conclude that there will be a moderately effective debate about RGTs. Some people will see no point in deliberation, but many will see the building blocks for a conversation. Those who can reach across a divide can be intermediaries in any discussion between those who truly do lack a shared language.

The percentage of people who share discourse across the divide cannot be precisely measured. A high estimate would come from the survey, which shows, for example, that 77 percent of non–pro-lifer, relative proponents of RGTs also use the meaningful suffering discourse. The optimistic interpretation here is that a very high percentage of the non–pro-lifers is familiar with this discourse and can at least imagine using it for some discussion about RGT. However, nowhere near this percentage of people use this discourse on their own in the in-depth interviews, presumably because, unlike the survey, we don't prompt them to use it. Nonetheless, the fact that a good number did, combined with the high number in the survey who could at least recognize the discourse as something they have used before, suggests there is the basis of conversation across the divide.

Moreover, the relief of suffering discourse is nearly universally shared and could be used for the basis of a conversation. Of course, I have shown that people use this discourse in different situations, but nearly everyone uses it for something and, more importantly, it is pervasively used to discuss human genetic engineering for cystic fibrosis. This is another strand that deliberation in the public sphere can be built on.

In the introduction I also discussed how the use of religious discourse in an RGT debate could dissuade people from deliberation because they will fear a lack of shared language. In chapter 7, I examined this closely and found that the religious nature of debates is not likely to dissuade people from debating.

An Improved Model for Understanding Effective Debates and Cultural Conflict

The culture wars' perspective claims that certain debates in the public sphere are polarized and unresolvable because of the religious nature of the debates and either the perception or actual lack of shared discourses with which to discuss social issues. In this perspective, the balkanization by discourse occurs because people talk about essentially all social issues using the same discourse, albeit an extremely abstract discourse, like "there is transcendent moral authority." Since the same discourse is used to oppose abortion, homosexuality, prayer in school, gender roles, and other social issues, like RGTs, people will perceive that talking about gender roles or RGTs is like talking about abortion or homosexuality, which is talked about with an uncompromising, nonuniversal discourse. People who are pro-choice then will not want to—and would not even be able to—deliberate about abortion with those who are pro-life. People on both sides of the homosexuality issue would also not deliberate and, recognizing that the same ultimate discourse is used for the homosexuality debate as the abortion debate. This is a model of total communication breakdown in the public sphere over social issues, which is exactly what Hunter's model predicted. Wars, after all, do not lend themselves to discussion, compromise, or the acknowledgment of similarities between the warring parties.

Scholars have rejected this model of cultural conflict as too sweeping, but without replacing it with a model that can be used to explain the conflict that we *do* see in debates in the public sphere. Retaining the theoretical presumption that a shared language is necessary to have a conversation in the public sphere, I developed a more specific model based on other scholars' theories that looks for shared discourse at a level much closer to the issue itself. All social issues are not assumed to be in two metadomains defined by an extremely abstract discourses like "moral authority comes from a transcendent source," but rather social issues are in distinct domains defined by the discourses that are directly used to talk about that issue. Moreover, in the culture wars model all social issues have the same degree of similarity; in my model they differ in similarity by the degree to which they have shared discourses. For example, given the discourses I have identified for the "opposition to genetic control" domain, unlike Hunter I would say that the issue of gender roles is essentially unrelated. Of course, people opposed to most RGTs also may be opposed to liberal gender roles, but critically it will not be for the same reasons—opening the possibility of deliberation with people who make opposing claims about one of these issues. My theoretical perspective also provides the answers to some unresolved questions in the debate about cultural conflict in the public sphere.

Understanding the Lack of Foot Soldiers in the Culture War

While the studies of ordinary people have found little evidence of increased polarization in attitudes toward social issues, these studies and others do suggest that the people who are more involved with the mediating institutions of the public sphere *are* polarized, decreasingly agreeing about social issues and generally lacking shared discourses with which to discuss these issues.[17] For example, members of Congress are much more polarized by party than they have been in the past, and the elites in social movement organizations are polarized—not many organizations are dedicated to promoting the "mushy middle" on social issues.[18] Media pundits and journalists also are polarized, with National Public Radio on one end and Fox News on the other. In short, people in mediating institutions in the public sphere are better described with Hunter's model than with my model.

A lack of shared discourses in the mediating institutions without a similar lack in the general public is puzzling, but can be understood by looking at the difference between the models. It has long been noted, starting at least with political scientist Phillip Converse in 1964, that social elites have stronger ideologies—organizing systems for their opinions.[19] "Ideology" is the political scientists' term for Hunter's worldview, and those more involved with political debates have more coherent and structured worldviews.[20] For people involved with debating these issues regularly, political scientists have shown that you can predict a person's position on abortion by his or her position on homosexuality and so on. "Individuals who are more familiar with the political world are more likely to develop ideologically-structured attitudes and perceptions," write two political scientists.[21]

In my model, the reason that people deeply involved with debates in the public sphere approximate Hunter's model—with all the negative ramifications—is precisely that they are debating with elite opponents who also organize their positions and discourses into worldviews. They are exposed enough to their opponents that, at some level of conservation that would be reached in time, there is indeed a lack of shared language at an abstract level. As I have shown, ordinary people tend to not organize their discourses and positions on issues into such rigid worldviews; for them there is no "culture war" on most issues.

Understanding Why the Abortion Debate Does Not Lead to Widespread Violence

Although there has been sporadic violence, such as the murder of doctors who provide abortion, there has not been widespread violence or even social conflict over culture wars issues. By and large, there has been no second American civil war, as some had predicted.[22]

I think the reason is that conflict would only ensue if people came to see their opponents as totally foreign. The nightmare scenario in the culture wars perspective is that people who are pro-life and pro-choice would have no shared language with which to discuss *any* issue. They would find that they used different discourses to talk about abortion, RGTs, homosexuality, prayer in school, gender roles, and on and on. Lacking anything that they had in common, they would come to see the other as totally foreign and as a potential threat to their view of the world. It is easy to demonize people we perceive as having nothing in common with us. Indeed, it is obvious that demonization of opponents is required before people can be convinced to kill them. For the Nazis, Jews and Roma were essentially a different species.

But, as I have shown, the pro-lifers and non–pro-lifers, while talking differently about abortion, often used the same discourse to talk about RGTs, which I have also shown to be an extremely similar issue to abortion. While they might agree to disagree about abortion for cystic fibrosis, many of them would find that they talked about sperm sorting and human genetic engineering the same way and probably came to the same conclusion. If I found that the same discourses were used on the RGT issue that is so similar to an issue with fundamental disagreement, it would be even more likely for people to use the same discourses on more distant issues from abortion like homosexuality or gender roles. Sharing some discourses, they would not see each other as foreign, but would see the other as someone who takes a reasonable position on many issues. Social conflict then would be less likely.

If there is little actual conflict over abortion, except among elites, we can probably also expect that there would not be conflict over RGTs among the ordinary citizens, given the shared discourses. Granted, with the data in this book I cannot evaluate the possibility of a secular versus religious culture war, but the percentage of Americans who are entirely divorced from religious discourses remains fairly small. Moreover, in the more theoretical culture wars model, the religious liberals we interviewed are in an opposing worldview from the religious conservatives, so I am accurately depicting at least the theoretical account of culture wars.[23]

A Solution to the Irreconcilable Abortion Debate?

In a review of recent research on attitudes toward abortion, political scientists Ted Jelen and Clyde Wilcox finish on a speculative note, writing that

> it will be interesting to track changes in the sources and distribution of abortion attitudes, and attitudes toward related issues, as questions of biotechnology (including variations on human cloning) become increasingly prominent in public discourse. As different values choices come into play (e.g. the intrinsic value of potential human life versus possible health benefits for living humans), and as different vested interests are created, it is difficult to imagine that abortion politics will not be transformed in some very basic ways [which has] the potential to create moral and political realignments in abortion discourse.[24]

Jelen and Wilcox do not provide a mechanism for how a debate about what they call biotechnology and variations on human cloning (which I would call RGTs) would transform the abortion debate. This is understandable because there is no theoretical tradition of which I am aware that would posit a mechanism. However, if the theoretical model I have developed here is accurate, and given my specific findings of the relationship between discourse about abortion and RGTs, we can see how the emergence of an RGT debate may change the abortion debate by decreasing the use of uncompromisable discourses.

First consider the pro-life side. As shown in the introduction, many pro-life organizations are already trying to create a broader issue domain that includes abortion and RGTs. I show that this domain already exists for pro-lifers—those who use the embryonic life discourse—who I would consider to be the natural constituency of the pro-life movement. If the RGT debate grows, people are going to be using more of the three discourses, raising them to prominence as a way to talk not only about RGTs but also about abortion for fetal defects, transforming the discourses that might otherwise have been used by pro-lifers. Given a fixed amount of words to utter about abortion, this would mean less use of the embryonic life discourse.

More critically, if the pro-life organizations adapt their claims to those the ordinary pro-lifers already use, they will produce educational materials and media messages that basically follow what is shown on the left side of figure 3. However, scholars of social movements have identified a tendency for domain expansion to result in more unified and more abstract discourses.[25] There will be pressures to not rely on four discourses but to come up with one discourse, inevitably more abstract, that can be used for all of the issues. Examination of the discourse of the antiabortion organizations suggests they already have such a discourse they are trying to promote to unify the opposition to abortion and to genetic control domains—that all these issues are "sanctity of life" issues. "Sanctity" of life is much more abstract than "not killing" life. Indeed, "sanctity" encompasses both "not killing" and "not modifying," and I would argue that as a general proposition more abstract discourses are perceived to be less absolutist, if only because their meaning is not immediately understood. Of course, these organizations will continue to use discourses like embryonic life to talk about abortion when a woman does not want to be pregnant and meaningful suffering for human genetic engineering for enhancements, but to the extent that social movement organizations have a fixed amount of discourse they can produce, people would start associating abortion with the "sanctity of life" discourse instead of the "embryonic life" discourse. This is much less absolutist and does not sound like the "clash of absolutes" in the current abortion debate. Pro-choice people would then be less likely to perceive a discussion with a user of the "sanctity of life" discourse to be pointless, and thus it is more likely that a conversation would at least be started about abortion. This would lessen the polarization in the abortion debate.

The growth of a debate about RGTs would also lower the polarization in the abortion debate through another mechanism. The results of this study show that many people on both sides of the abortion debate use the same discourse—and reach the same conclusion—about enhancement RGTs. People on both sides of the abortion debate who are opposed to preimplantation genetic diagnosis for enhancement could then build from the three discourses to discuss abortion for fetal defect. The person on the pro-choice side does not at present use the three discourses to discuss abortion, but, as I have shown, these issues are extremely similar for many people. They could then have that discussion about abortion, across the supposed divide, about whether the three discourses under close examination in this book can be applied to abortion. Similarly, both sides use the discourse of relief of suffering, albeit for different RGTs, and the pro-choice person could have that conversation across the supposed divide by trying to convince the pro-lifer that preimplantation genetic diagnosis for health applications is analogous to human genetic engineering for health. In short, the availability of shared discourses on issues that I have demonstrated to be considered very similar to abortion increases the chance of a conversation about abortion which would, again, lessen polarization and transform the debate.

Open Questions in the New Culture Wars Debate

With this more specific theoretical apparatus in place, I see a number of additional research questions. The first item on the agenda would be to try to observe deliberation about issues in the public sphere. I have conducted an empirical study of how people talk about different issues, but the connection between these patterns of talk and the ability to talk with others is based on other scholars' theories and studies. Although some political scientists have created various deliberation experiments, they are not usually focused on whether people with different positions can effectively share their perspectives and reach a consensus. This research will probably have to occur using ethnographic case studies; therefore, the findings will be limited in the scope of their applicability, but with a number of studies we may see a pattern emerging.[26]

For the second item on the agenda, rather than presuming a discursive divide between the supporters and opponents of all social issues, let us instead map where the divide actually exists. Note that this is different from the existing literature which examines if people have patterns in their *conclusions* about social issues—whether those opposed to abortion are also opposed to homosexuality, egalitarian gender roles, and so on. It has been shown that there are moderate tendencies for conclusions to be grouped, but when the culture wars debate is recast as a question of the ability to deliberate in the public sphere, the question is whether people who reach opposite conclusions about an issue have the ability to deliberate about these conclusions. More critically, and for example, do people who reach different conclusions about homosexuality have more shared discourses compared to the degree of shared discourses on an issue like abortion? Then, even if the nation were perfectly evenly split on conclusions about both abortion and homosexuality, we would predict that homosexuality would have a more effective debate in the public sphere.

A third issue that will need closer examination is the difference between not knowing a discourse versus knowing a discourse but not using it. It seems likely that the issues where there is a lack of deliberation, like abortion, are ones where the discourse used by one side (e.g., embryonic life) is not used for any situation by the people on the other side. To be precise, the people on the other side may know the discourse and be able to repeat it to you, but do not "believe in it"—they do not use it for any argument about any situation. For other discourses, like "reduction of suffering," everyone uses it for some situation at some point in their lives. It seems likely that the use of discourses that are used by both sides of a debate, albeit for different situations, would result in more deliberation. But, this remains an empirical question.

Go Deliberate

I believe that something important can be learned from deliberating issues with people with whom you do not agree, even if you never compromise your position. This is particularly true on issues that are new—where people have not thought through all the implications. A debate about RGTs will happen, and I have described the initial position of the religious community toward RGTs. However, there will be pressures toward an ineffective debate. Because antiabortion organizations are talking first, we may perceive that we should not try to discuss RGTs. But, if people try to deliberate, they will find they have more to talk about than they think. What is certain is that we do not want to just stumble forward toward the future without having a conversation about what we as a society want to do about RGTs. We can all agree that an effective debate about RGTs would be healthy for the human future.

Methodological Appendix

Interview Data

To be able to see what exactly this book represents, it is important to be clear about the exact methodology that I used. As usual, methodological decisions are trade-offs based on the research goals and available resources. I felt it was imperative to have long interviews, between one and two hours, which precluded using telephones. This then excluded using a truly random sample of religious people in the United States, because I could not afford to fly a research assistant to each randomly selected person in the United States. I decided that the interviews would have to be grouped geographically, and I would send a research assistant to each location.

Since I wanted the interviewees to match the distribution of religious affiliations in the United States, I decided to find congregations in each geographic location that were firmly in the religious tradition for which I was looking. I wanted to recruit people from congregations that were stereotypically mainline Protestant, evangelical, and so on.

I could have used random sampling at this point. I could have gone to a phone book in a community and classified all the congregations by tradition. Since we would have been, at most, selecting one congregation from each of the religious traditions in each geographic location, we could have randomly sampled one congregation from each tradition. The danger here is that we were only selecting a few congregations in each geographic location, and never more than one of the same type to ensure geographic diversity. If we had randomly sampled congregations with this "low N" per location strategy, we could have ended up with a congregation that is very idiosyncratic to the larger tradition. Without the "large N" to marginalize idiosyncrasy, we could end up with a Pentecostal mainline Protestant church or a nontraditional evangelical congregation that is actually fundamentalist. We needed a method to identify congregations that were appropriate representatives of each tradition.

Local Expert Study

In spring 2003, I hired eight research assistants who were either located across the country or who were willing to live for a while in a specific location. Each research assistant was assigned two geographic locations. Beginning in the first location, each research assistant conducted an informal expert poll to identify congregations. They called well-placed religious leaders, such as the directors of ecumenical organizations and local religious coalitions; and congregational leaders, as well as academics who had studied these communities, and asked them: "If I had just moved to town, and I had said to you that I was mainline Protestant and looking for a church home, where would you tell me to visit?" Then, the question was repeated for each religious tradition that I was trying to identify in that geographic area.

We planned on calling ten to fifteen leaders in each geographic location and aggregating their responses. Obviously, in some towns it only took one call to identify the one Catholic church or Jewish synagogue. In other towns, we relied on particularly knowledgeable people to make our task easier. But, most often, it took a good number of calls to start forming a consensus. The most frequently mentioned congregation in each category became the target of our recruitment effort.

What can we expect to get from this? We can expect to have identified congregations that these experts think of as embodying these traditions. They will not send a mainline Protestant to a Presbyterian church that, while in a mainline denomination, is more classically evangelical, or send an evangelical to a mainline church. What will occur with this method is that the congregations will be more "middle of the road" in these traditions. For example, when asking about evangelical congregations, we were never referred to a Jehovah's Witness or Mormon congregation, because these are not classically thought of as evangelical Protestant. We were never sent to a Seventh Day Adventist congregation. Rather, we were sent to congregations that are the guardians of the traditions embodied in the labels. In my evaluation of the congregations that we targeted I was rarely surprised. I spoke with many of the leaders of these congregations, and the conversations confirmed that we were on target. Other materials confirmed this conclusion. The Web sites of mainline Protestant congregations showed pipe organs, children's and handbell choirs, service opportunities, and middle of the road, somewhat intellectual sermons. Nontraditional evangelical congregations were obvious because they are so different, with guitars, projection monitors, praise bands, plays, and so on, with sermons focused on the immediate experiences of the members. People had no problem with Pentecostals: referring us to Assemblies of God and Church of God (Cleveland, TN) congregations. I believe the respondents had a little harder time distinguishing between fundamentalists and traditional evangelicals, with more variation in their responses. However, the congregations we targeted were clearly on target.

With this method we can also expect a bias toward more functional congregations and toward larger congregations that will be known by more people. This would be a problem if we had a theory for why people at smaller and less functional congregations would have different views on these issues. There is no obvious reason why this would be the case.

The decision to concentrate on which geographic areas also was a bit of an art. The first criterion was the region of the country, because it is quite plausible that members of a religion in one region are slightly different from another. While I do not expect large differences, it seems the safer strategy than to have all the interviews in one place such as Southern California. I decided to conduct interviews in California, the Northeast, the Midwest, the South, and the Southeast. More precise geographic placement was next based on the urban-rural dimension, where I strived to have a mix of places represented. Beyond that, location was based on the purely pragmatic issue of where the best research assistants I could find in each region were living, trying to avoid having them drive more than thirty minutes each way for their interviews. Within thirty minutes of each research assistant was a wide selection of neighborhoods, cities, and towns from which to select. Each research assistant conducted research near their primary location and then conducted the expert study by phone at their secondary location, later living in the secondary location to conduct the interviews. At this point, I became more strategic as possible to try to make the interviews as representative of religion in the United States.

It is often said that Sunday morning at 11:00 a.m. is the most segregated hour in American life. In light of this, sampling by congregation will result in a high degree of racial homogeneity within each congregation. Similarly, geographic segregation by race, ethnicity, and class is very strong in the United States; thus, the decision of which geographic area to focus on is simultaneously a decision of what race, ethnicity, or class that you would like the respondents to have. At this point, I wanted diversity in race or ethnicity (white/black/Hispanic), class, and cosmopolitanism (city/suburb/small town).

To select a geographic interview location based purely on race or class would have resulted in too much concentration of interviews. At most I needed interviewees from two Hispanic Catholic churches. If we were to select East Los Angeles (where it could be guaranteed that all respondents were Hispanic), we would be unsure whether we were describing a Hispanic sample or a sample of Southern Californians. To avoid this problem as best as possible, given the limited numbers of interviews, we focused on geographic areas that were only segregated at the neighborhood level. Cities, for example, are racially and economically mixed—although still expected to be segregated at the congregational level.

How We Found Our Interviewees

Either I or the research assistants then approached the religious leader of the target congregation and asked for their cooperation. Leaders were asked to produce the names of six members who would be "good at giving their opinions on the issue," and six more people were selected randomly from the membership list. For the "selected" names, religious leaders were asked to give us names of men and women, and younger and older people. Two "selected" and two "random" members would be interviewed. If a congregation refused to participate, we would move to the next most mentioned congregation in the category. I examined each target congregation to confirm that it was truly in the category for which we were looking before having it approached by the research assistant.

While identifying the target congregations in each geographic location, I also had conducted ten pilot interviews using a snowball sample methodology in San Diego County during winter and early spring 2003, continuously reworking the interview guide (these are not analyzed in this book). This became the first interview guide used by the research assistants.

With his or her list of people to interview in the primary location, each research assistant interviewed two respondents and then stopped. These interviews were transcribed and then I evaluated them. In May 2003, we had a meeting where we discussed the interviews that had been conducted thus far, looking over transcripts and listening to snippets of interviews. We changed question wording and discussed various follow-up probes that could have been used in particular situations. After the meeting, researchers continued with their interviewing.

How Many of Each Type of Congregation?

The number of interviews per religious tradition would be influenced by the size of the group in relation to the population of the United States, while retaining enough cases for meaningful analysis. There were 180 completed interviews. I wanted to make a comparison to nonreligious people, so I decided a priori that one-fifth of the interviews would be with people who are not members of religious congregations. The remaining four-fifths of the interviews (145 interviews) were allocated according to the size of the religious group among religious attenders in the United States.

An exception to this rule was interviews with Jews. By strict proportion in the U.S. population, I would have interviewed 2.7 Jews. As I explained in the introduction, I felt it important to have enough Jews in the sample to legitimately be able to say something about the differences in views between Christians and Jews. I planned on conducting twenty interviews with Jews, spread throughout the various traditions, and ended with seventeen. Of those Jews who are members of synagogues, 41 percent belong to a Reform temple, 41 percent to a Conservative synagogue, and 18 percent to an Orthodox synagogue.[1] To roughly approximate this statistic, we interviewed eight members from the Conservative movement and nine members of either the Reform or Reconstructionist movements.[2] Although I had planned to have four interviews with members of a modern Orthodox synagogue, the one congregation was scheduled near the end of the project, and when they declined to participate at the last minute, the other research assistants could not offer a substitute because they were in locations without an Orthodox synagogue (e.g., a rural area in the Northeast). There are obviously not enough interviews with members of the different traditions to make claims of differences *within* Judaism, but to compare Judaism to the other traditions in the United States.

While mainline Protestants can be found in most Protestant denominations, usually they are thought of as clustering within a number of historically mainline denominations. The six largest mainline denominations are the United Methodist Church, the Episcopal Church, the Presbyterian Church (USA), the United Church of Christ, the Evangelical Lutheran Church in America, and the American Baptist Churches.[3] In 1998 they had twenty-two million members.[4] Chaves, Giesel, and Tsitsos found that 23 percent of those *attending churches* in the United States were members of the six largest mainline denominations.[5] So, I tried to make 22 percent of our church member interviews be interviews of mainline Protestants (thirty-two interviews) and ended with 24 percent (thirty-four interviews). Our method of interviewing local experts resulted in the congregation functioning as the stereotypical "mainline" congregation being United Methodist, United Church of Christ, Presbyterian Church (USA), or another traditional mainline denomination. These denominations are almost purely white; thus, we made no effort to find black or Hispanic mainline churches.

Chaves, Giesel, and Tsitsos also found that 25 percent of attenders were Catholic.[6] So, we attempted to have 22 percent of the church member interviews be with Catholics. Catholicism in the United States is very racially diverse, if not within congregations, at least between them. The major diversity is ethnicity, with between 30 and 38 percent of all U.S. Catholics being Hispanic.[7] In some areas, there are large numbers of Vietnamese, Filipinos, and other immigrant groups to diversify the earlier immigrants from Ireland and central Europe. We wanted to interview ten Hispanic Catholics of the thirty-two Catholic interviews. We ended with forty-one interviews of Catholics—29 percent of all the interviews of congregation members—with six being Hispanics.

Chaves, Giesel, and Tsitsos found that approximately 50 percent of attenders were "other Protestants," a very heterogeneous group more conservative than mainline Protestants, which would roughly be categorized as evangelicals and fundamentalists or "conservative Protestants."[8] Having "taken" a few interviews from mainline Protestants and Catholics to make room for the 14 percent of the member sample devoted to examining Judaism, I "took" the rest from conservative Protestantism, hoping to have 42 percent of the interviews come from this group (sixty interviews). We ended with 35 percent of the interviews from conservative Protestants, and fifty interviews in total.

Conservative Protestantism is a very heterogeneous category, and I wanted to make sure to roughly capture the diversity of these more conservative Protestants. Here we have to remind ourselves that great precision is not possible because I grouped interviews by congregation, resulting in our approaching twelve congregations in total (to obtain the fifty interviews). Since most African Americans are theologically conservative, it is here that I looked to find black congregations, targeting eight interviews with members of two black evangelical congregations. Pentecostalism is also an important component of evangelicalism, so I targeted three congregations, resulting in eleven more interviews. The largest group of interviewees was what I call "traditional evangelicals," such as Southern Baptists, Nazarenes, and the Christian and Missionary Alliance. We targeted five congregations, resulting in nineteen interviews. Although the media and public discourse often calls all conservative Protestants "fundamentalists," actual fundamentalists are a small subset of conservative Protestants. We interviewed eight members of two fundamentalist churches.

The remaining twelve interviews (from three congregations) were from what we called "nontraditional evangelicals." I felt it important to at least tap into this growing segment of evangelicalism, given that the theology and way of interacting with the broader community is so different for this group. These are churches in the seeker mold or, similarly, from the Calvary Chapel, Vineyard, and Willow Creek format.[9] When conducting our local expert survey, we specified what we meant here by asking for the names of congregations where there was a nontraditional worship service, songs on overhead projectors, informal dress, or like Calvary Chapel, Willow Creek, or a "seeker" church. We ended with a Vineyard congregation, and two congregations explicitly using a "seeker" model that are loosely affiliated with traditional evangelical denominations. As our method would suggest, these were very clearly different from traditional evangelical churches (e.g., projection televisions, plays instead of sermons, and greeters in Hawaiian shirts).

Nonreligious Interviews

I also wanted to compare the interviews of the members of congregations with those who are not religiously committed. I am not interested in the small number of atheists in this country. Rather, I am interested in that fairly large portion of the United States that believes in God and was perhaps raised in a particular tradition, but does not participate in organized religious activities.

Obviously identifying people who are not members of religious congregations requires a different strategy. The strategy is also not obvious, given that there are no organizations of the "religiously uninvolved." Therefore, for this part of the project, we relied on a purposive, quota sample of people who do not attend religious services. We interviewed roughly equal numbers of men and women, and younger and older people. We interviewed people with a diversity of educational experiences and occupations. In each geographic location, we only needed to interview between two and four of these people; thus, the research assistant in that area was assigned particular types of nonreligious people to find.

The "nonreligious" interviewees were identified through one of two network methods. In one, we would ask the religious interviewees at the end of the interview whether they had a friend, family member, coworker, or anyone they knew who did not attend religious services and who might be willing to sit for an interview. For a second method, we would start with personal contacts in the region and then identify the type of person in question and secure the interview. When soliciting the interview, we would confirm that they fit the category for which we were looking. There is no obvious difference in the responses of the people identified using these two methods. The interview guide for the religious respondents follows this appendix. The guide for the secular respondents was slightly different—primarily removing questions about religious practice that were not relevant.

Analyzing the Interview Data

The interviews were transcribed and then input into the qualitative data analysis program called NVivo. I then interpretively coded the data. I tried to not have my preconceptions about how people from different religious traditions would respond bias my coding of the data, so I would begin coding after the initial part of the interview, when they identified themselves religiously. Of course, with some respondents, their religious tradition is evident from the way that they talk about anything, but I did the best I could to initially look at each interview in a more neutral way.

Survey Data

I use a 4,800-respondent Internet-based survey, commissioned by the Genetics and Public Policy Center, that is nationally representative of the American public aged eighteen years or older. Knowledge Networks, a survey research firm, has developed a panel of respondents who are given free Internet access for their homes, which they use for both personal use and to answer occasional surveys. The sample is representative because the panelists are selected through a standard random-digit dial procedure and are given the computer equipment and online access. The method has been studied extensively and has been demonstrated to be as representative as random digit dialing.[10] Papers using Knowledge Networks surveys have been published in *JAMA, Health Services Research*, the *Journal of Personality and Social Psychology*, and other prestigious publications. This survey, fielded in March 2004, had a 73 percent response rate, resulting in 4,834 completed interviews. Similar to most surveys, this one is weighted to reflect the demographic distribution of the U.S. population aged 18 years and older. To assuage concerns that religious affiliation might not be accurately represented in the study, I compared the percentage claiming each religious tradition in the Knowledge Networks study with identically worded religious affiliation questions in a random-digit dial study.[11] I found that the percentages were within 2.1 percent of each other for each religious group. Questions and the coding of the responses are described in the text.

Religious Respondent Interview Guide

(I) Informed Consent Statement and Explanation. Audiotape Consent Signing

(II) Introduction

Read: "As you probably know, our genes determine the details of our bodies. For example, there are genes for skin color, height, and some that can make you get certain diseases. Half of our children's genes come from the father and half from the mother. In recent years it has become possible to not only *know* what genetic traits you are passing down to your children, but in some cases it is possible to decide that your children will or will not get certain genes. To take the simplest example, a couple who knows that they have the gene that causes the disease called cystic fibrosis can decide to adopt their children instead. To take an example that is not yet possible, scientists think that in the future parents will be able to directly change the genes of the baby right after conception to give them genes the parents want to give them.

I know that you may not have thought a lot about these issues before today. That is fine. In fact, we do not want to talk with experts on this topic, but we want to talk to average Americans to see what they think. So don't worry if your answers to my questions seem 'off the cuff.' Everyone's answers on these questions are 'off the cuff.' It's OK to be thinking through the issues while talking.

This project has nothing to do with your church or synagogue. They will not hear the interview or see transcripts of it. We will not be reporting to them. We received the names of twelve people from the congregation, and are only interviewing four of these people, so the people at the congregation will not know whether we have interviewed you or one of the other people."

(III) Demographics

Before beginning, I need some basic information about you so I can compare your responses to similar people.

QUESTION (Q): Do you have any family members or close friends who have genetic disease, or who have had children with genetic disease?
[IF so, ask what it is.]

Q: If you or a spouse are currently pregnant or have ever lost a pregnancy due to a genetic problem with the baby, or if you had faced a particularly emotional decision regarding pregnancy, you may not want to continue with the interview.

Q: What is your occupation?

Q: How many children? How old are they?

Q: Are you Catholic, Protestant, Jewish, or something else?

[FOR PROTESTANTS]: When it comes to your religious identity, would you say you are a fundamentalist, evangelical, mainline, or liberal Protestant, or do none of these describe you?

[FOR CATHOLICS]: When it comes to your religious identity, would you say you are a traditional, moderate, or liberal Catholic, or do none of these describe you?

[FOR JEWS]: Would you consider yourself to be Orthodox, Conservative, Reform, or none of the above?

Q: How often do you attend religious services? [For Protestants, if you don't already know: "Which specific denomination is that?"]

Q: In addition, do you go to adult education classes, Sunday school, Bible studies, prayer groups, or similar events at the congregation?

Q: What is the most advanced educational degree that you have? What was your major?

[Q PRELIMINARY QUESTION I (PR I)]: I have a number of hypothetical scenarios. Before I get to them, I have one quick preliminary question. Children of parents who work hard often work hard themselves. Do you think that there is a gene that causes people to work hard?

[PROBE: If "no": "What makes people work hard then?" If they say some mixed response: "How much of working hard can be explained by the gene and how much by how they were raised by their parents?"]

(IV) Introduction to Scenarios

Now I'm going to describe different hypothetical couples who are planning to have children and ask you for your opinions about each situation. These are made-up situations. There are no right or wrong answers, I just want to find out your opinion.

[Q SCENARIO 1 (S1): Screening for cystic fibrosis]

READ: "Here is the situation. A friend of yours, Mary, just found out that she and her husband Mark both have the gene that causes cystic fibrosis. Since Mary and Mark each have only one copy of the gene, they aren't sick, they are only what are called 'carriers.' Cystic fibrosis is a genetic disease where children's lungs do not work properly, and the average child with cystic fibrosis dies by the time they are thirty years old from lung problems. If they were to have a child, there is a one in four chance that their child would get both copies of the gene, and then would be sick with cystic fibrosis."

Q: They really want to have children of their own, but are worried about this disease. What should they do?

[Q SCENARIO 2 (S2): Amniocentesis for cystic fibrosis]

READ: "How about if this story had been different. What if Mary was already two months pregnant when she found out about these genes? There is a one in four chance that their child would get both copies of the gene, and would be sick with cystic fibrosis. The doctor gives them these options: (1) they can wait until fifteen weeks into the pregnancy and test the fetus to see if it has the disease and then decide whether to have an abortion, or (2) not test the fetus and see what happens."

Q: What should they do? Why?

[Q SCENARIO 3 (S3): Preimplantation genetic diagnosis (PGD) for cystic fibrosis]

READ: "Imagine another couple named Bob and Barbara. They have found out that they each have the gene for cystic fibrosis *before* they started to try to have a baby. They know that there is a one in four chance that their children will have cystic fibrosis. They visit a doctor who tells them of a technique called preimplantation genetic diagnosis. This is a new technology that I did not even know about until I started working on this project, so I'll explain it to you. What this means is that the doctor will collect six eggs from Barbara and sperm from Bob and mix them together in his laboratory. This is often called 'in vitro fertilization' or what the media calls making "test-tube babies." After each of the fertilized eggs have developed into an early embryo made up of eight cells, the doctor will remove a cell from each embryo and test it to see which embryos are disease free. Then he can implant the disease-free embryos in Barbara's uterus to try to start a pregnancy. Although no one knows for sure, taking the one cell off of the embryo doesn't seem to cause problems for any baby that results. With this method, they are sure they won't have a baby that has cystic fibrosis."

Q: Should they use this way of making a baby?

Q: Is this better than the situation I just told you about, where they tested the fetus in the womb and maybe would have an abortion?

Q: Is there anything that makes you uncomfortable about this technique? Anything else?

[Q SCENARIO 4 (S4): PGD for Alzheimer's disease]

READ: "Tina and Tim have a similar situation. But the issue is not cystic fibrosis. Many members of Tim's family have been diagnosed with Alzheimer's disease very early in life, around age fifty. Tina and Tim would like to make sure their child doesn't have the gene for early Alzheimer's disease. It turns out that they can use this preimplantation genetic diagnosis technology, the same technique we were just discussing, to look for embryos that have the Alzheimer gene."

Q: Should they do this?

Q: What makes this different than the situation with cystic fibrosis, if anything?

[Q S4A: PGD for deafness]

READ: "What if the test was not for a gene for cystic fibrosis or Alzheimer's, but rather for a gene that causes children to be born deaf?

Q: "Would this make a difference in whether you think it's appropriate to use this technology? Why?"

[Q S4B: PGD for obesity]

READ: "What if this test was not for cystic fibrosis, Alzheimer's, or deafness, but a gene for obesity? A gene like this isn't guaranteed to make someone obese, just make them more likely to be obese."

Q: Would this make a difference in whether you think it's appropriate to use this technology? Why?

[Q S4C: PGD for intelligence]

READ: "What if it was not for cystic fibrosis or Alzheimer's, but rather they were looking for the embryo that had the best genes for intelligence?"

Q: Would this make a difference in whether you think it's appropriate to use PGD? Why?

[POSSIBLE PROBE IF THEY ARE OPPOSED: "Some people would say it would be better if people could make their children smarter. What would you say to them?"]

Q: Should we regulate *which* genetic traits can be tested for in embryos? How would you decide what genetic traits to regulate?

[PROBE, IF "YES": "Some people would say that they have a right to control what their children are like. What would you say to that?"]

[Q S5: Sex selection]

READ: "Another couple is named Andy and Ann. They do not have any known genetic diseases, but they already have two boys and they really want to have a girl in their family. There are a number of options available to them to try to have a girl: (1) Ann can just become pregnant "the old fashioned way" and see what happens; (2) They could adopt a girl; (3) Ann could become pregnant and then test the fetus for its sex, and have an abortion if it is a boy."

Q: Which of these three should they do?

READ: "A method that they could use is preimplantation genetic diagnosis, where they would look at each of the embryos and only implant a girl embryo."

Q: Do you think they should do this?

[Q S5A: Sperm sorting]

READ: "Another method they could use is called 'sperm sorting.' Here, all they have to do it to take Andy's sperm and sort it into male and female sperm. Only the female sperm are put inside of Ann's uterus with the hope that she would become pregnant."

Q: Do you think they should do this? Is this better than the other methods?

Q: What would be good and bad effects on society if this sperm-sorting technology were available to anyone who wanted to use it? [If they say gender imbalance, then say, "Any other problems?"]

Q: Is there anything about this that makes you uncomfortable?

Q: [For those who see bad effects] Should this technique of sperm sorting be legal?

Q: Do you think that if Andy and Ann used this sperm sorting technique to produce a girl, they would think of that child any differently than their other children?

[Q s6: Germline engineering]

READ: "I am now going to tell you about a technology that is not yet available. Now let's talk about Sam and Sue. They have two children, both of whom have cystic fibrosis. Lets say that doctor has perfected a new technique. Not only can he test for diseases, he can fix the genes in fertilized eggs to remove the chance that any baby would have cystic fibrosis. If Sam and Sue have a child in this way, not only will this child be free of this gene, but so would that child's children, and that child's grandchildren and so on. It would remove this gene from their family tree for good."

Q: Should they do this?

Q: Should we allow this in our country?

[Q s6A: Human genetic engineering (HGE) for obesity]

Q: Would you think differently about Sue and Sam's situation if the gene they wanted to change was for obesity?

[Q s6B: HGE for Intelligence]

Q: Would your opinion change about Sue and Sam's situation if they wanted to use this technique to give their baby, as well as all of their descendants, more intelligence?

[Q s6c: HGE with shot]

Q: How about if the technology were different. What if instead of changing the genes in fertilized eggs, doctors could give Sam a shot that changes the genes in Sam's sperm so that any babies that he fathers will be free of the cystic fibrosis gene. Would this make a difference in what you thought of using this technology?

Q: If they made their child more intelligent, do you think that Sam and Sue would raise that child any differently than their other children?

[Q s7: Cloning]

READ: "Finally, lets talk about Donna and David. I assume you have heard about human cloning. This is where you make a baby with the exact same genes as somebody else. What would be done is that a cell from somebody's skin is put into a woman's egg, and then made to start growing. The embryo that grows from this event is put into a woman's uterus and grows into a baby. Donna and David want their child to excel in life, so they have decided to clone a person that they both really admire."

Q: Should they do this?

Q: Would you consider this cloned child to be just as human as everyone else? Why?

[PROBE: "Some would disagree and say that they are not human. What would you say to someone who said that?"]

Q: Would this cloned child have a soul?

(V) Effects on Society at Large

[*Asterisk indicates most important questions in final five sections, if time becomes limited.*]

Now, I'm going to ask you some general questions:

* Q SOCIETY-AT-LARGE QUESTION I (SL1): In your responses to the previous questions, you seemed to want families to avoid having children with genetic diseases. I know it seems like a silly question, but could you tell me, in your own words, why we want to stop people from getting genetic disease?

* Q SL2: I have another silly question. Can you tell me, in your own words, what a disease is?

Q SL3: Do you know what the word eugenics means?

IF "YES": Can you tell me what it means, in your own words?

IF "NO": Eugenics is the attempt to improve the so-called "genetic quality" of the people who live in a country.

Q SL4: In the past, governments have promoted eugenic programs. Are you worried that when these technologies become widely available governments will encourage eugenic programs to "improve" the genetic characteristics of their citizens?

Q SL5: Would you agree or disagree with the following statement: "There is no invention or technology that is totally good or bad, it depends upon how people use it."

* Q SL6: If you knew a couple who were facing one of those difficult decisions we discussed earlier, who would be the most important person they should talk to before making their decision? Why?

Q: Who else should they talk to? Why?

(VI) Religion

* Q RELIGION QUESTION I (R1): Now I want to ask some questions about religion. Does any passage in the Bible, other religious teaching, or religious concept come to mind as being particularly important for

understanding the issues we have been talking about? ("Imagine you are teaching a Sunday school class on these topics, and you want to put a quote from the Bible or some other religious teaching on the blackboard.") Many people we interview do not come up with anything here, because they haven't thought enough about the issue before today, so don't worry if you cannot come up with anything.

* Q R2: Can you tell me, in your own words, what the first chapter in the book of Genesis says?

Q: Is this passage relevant to the issues we have been discussing? How?

* Q R3: Are you familiar with the Biblical account of the Tower of Babel? [Gen 11:1–9]. Can you tell me what it is?

[If people give some version of a response, do not correct them, but accept it and move on. If they have no idea, tell them it is a short and minor story in the book of Genesis and summarize it very briefly.]

Q: Is this passage relevant to the issues we have been discussing? How?

* Q R4: Are you familiar with the book of Job? What is the main message of the book of job? Is the book of Job relevant to the issues we have been discussing? How?

* Q R5: In the books of Matthew, Mark, and Luke, the stories of Jesus healing many people's diseases is told.

Q: Are these stories of Jesus's healing ministry relevant to the issues we have been discussing? How?

Q R6: Did God create genetic diseases?

[PROBE IF "YES": Why did God create genetic diseases?]

[PROBE IF "NO": Where do you think they came from then?]

Q R7: What influence do you think your own religious beliefs have on your conclusions about these issues?

* Q R8: Does God want us to create these new technologies? Which ones?

* Q R9: The Bible says that humans were made in the image of God. Is this passage relevant to the issues we have been discussing?

Q: Are children produced through the technologies we have been discussing today made in the image of God?

* Q R10: Should the ability to change the genes of the human species be reserved for God?

* Q R11: What do you think the phrase, "We shouldn't play God," means?

Q R12: Are science and religion in conflict? Why?

Q: Can you give me an example of when they *do* conflict?

Q RI3: If God is the creator of the world and the life on it, are you comfortable with saying that humans are "co-Creators" with God in trying to heal diseases?

• Q RI4: Should we try to eliminate all of people's suffering?

(VII) Role of Religious Denomination/Tradition

* Q TRADITION QUESTION I (TI): Have you ever heard a sermon or had a Sunday school class that discussed any of these technologies? Have you ever heard a sermon or had a Sunday school class that discussed abortion?
* Q T2: Will you be looking to the leaders of your religious tradition or denomination to help you think through these issues in the future?
* Q T3: Do you think that your denomination (or movement) has an official position on these technologies?
Q: What do you think that it is?
Q: Do you think that denominations (or movements) should take official positions on issues like this?
Q: Should they try to influence the Congress to pass laws based upon these official positions?

(VI) The Nature of Public and Debate

* Q PUBLIC DEBATE QUESTION I (PI): I know what you think about these issues and the advice you would give. Do you think it should be legal for *other people* to change the genes of their children to make them more intelligent?
[PROBE: "What about parents? Some people would say they should decide."]
[PROBE: "Some people would say that this is the sort of thing that society should control. What would you say to them?"]
Q P2: Do you think that the scientists who are developing these technologies generally have the same values you do?
Q: What values should we keep in mind as we debate whether to use these technologies?
Q P3: There is a public debate about whether to allow these technologies. Some of this debate is about what we should teach to the youth of

America about these technologies, some of this debate is about what laws, if any, should regulate these technologies. Do you think that people who share your values will be influential in this debate?

[IF "NO": "Who do you think will be influential?"]

* Q P4: Imagine that we were going to have a meeting of ten people that would recommend which of these technologies would be allowed and under what circumstances. The decision the group reaches would be sent to the Congress to be considered as a possible law. What types of training or interest should the people have?

   [PROBE: What would the value of the input of [profession #1] be?]

   [PROBE: What would the value of the input of [profession #2] be?]

* Q P5: So, you are Catholic (or, _____), and you have your particularly Catholic way of thinking about these issues. Lets say that your next-door neighbor is from India, and they practice the Hindu religion, and they have a Hindu way of thinking about these issues. Lets also say that you are having a conversation with them about genetics. Should you explain your position on these issues using religious terms or secular terms?

Q: Is it possible to express your views accurately on these topics without discussing religious ideas?

Q P6: Many people have religious reasons to support or oppose these technologies. When debating these issues in public, should they use a nonreligious way of talking or can they use their religious way of talking to explain their position?

Q P7: Can you imagine some technology having to do with genetics and having children that you would want banned forever, no matter what the good consequences? What would that be?

(VII) Closing Statements

We are almost done.

* Q Closing Statement Question 1 (C1): [Hand card] When you think about all the issues that we have talked about today, which one of these words best summarizes your feelings. Or, you can pick a word that is not on the list. Or, you can talk about more than one if you want. Why?

* Q C2: Is there anything else that came to mind during the interview that you didn't get a chance to say that you want to mention?

* Q C3: We would like to compare what members of churches and synagogues say to people who are not particularly religious. Can you think of people know who might be willing to be interviewed for this project but who are not, to your knowledge, members of a church or synagogue?

Notes

Acknowledgments

1. John H. Evans, "Religious Belief, Perceptions of Human Suffering and Support for Reproductive Genetic Technology," *Journal of Health Politics, Policy and Law* 31, no. 6 (2006): 1047–74.

Chapter One

1. David Frum, "The Vanishing Republican Voter: Why Income Inequality is Destroying the G.O.P. Base," *New York Times* (Sunday Magazine), September 7, 2008, 51.

2. Francis Fukuyama, *Our Posthuman Future: Consequences of the Biotechnology Revolution* (New York: Farrar, Straus and Giroux, 2002).

3. Chorionic villi sampling has the same logic as amniocentesis, but occurs earlier in pregnancy. I do not discuss this RGT further because the moral issues are nearly identical with amniocentesis and it would have been much less familiar to the respondents.

4. These definitions are derived from the President's Council on Bioethics, *Beyond Therapy: Biotechnology and the Pursuit of Happiness* (Washington, DC: President's Council on Bioethics, 2003), 13. How to draw this distinction is an enormous debate in normative ethics, which primarily focuses on the meaning of the word "normal." For a summary of this debate, see John H. Evans and Cynthia E. Schairer, "Bioethics and Human Genetic Engineering," in *Handbook of Genetics and Society: Mapping the New Genomic Era*, ed. Paul Atkinson, Peter Glasner, and Margaret Lock (London: Routledge, 2009), 349–66; and Erik Parens, "Is Better Always Good? The Enhancement Project," in *Enhancing Human Traits: Ethical and Social Implications*, ed. Erik Parens (Washington, DC: Georgetown University Press, 1998), 1–28.

5. John Harris, "Who's afraid of a synthetic human?" *TimesOnline*, May 17, 2008.

6. John Harris, *Enhancing Evolution: The Ethical Case for Making Better People* (Princeton: Princeton University Press, 2007).

7. Human Genetics Commission members (http://www.hgc.gov.uk/client/content_wide.asp?ContentId=21).

8. Evans and Schairer, "Bioethics and Human Genetic Engineering."

9. Fiona Macrae. "The IVF embryo test that can detect 15,000 genetic diseases," *Daily Mail*, July 1, 2009.

10. Mark Henderson, "Gene Tests to Start Era of Baby-to-Order," *The Times (London)* June 26, 2004, 1.

11. Fiona Macrae, "Designer baby row erupts over embryo 'squint test'," *Daily Mail* (London), May 7, 2007; and Darshak M. Sanghavi, "Wanting babies like themselves, some parents choose genetic defects," *New York Times*, December 5, 2006, F1.

12. Douglas Almond and Lena Edlund, "Son-Biased Sex Ratios in the 2000 United States Census," *Proceedings of the National Academy of Sciences* 105, no. 15 (2008): 5681–82.

13. Gautam Naik, "A Baby, Please. Blond, Freckles—Hold the Colic," *Wall Street Journal Online*, February 12, 2009.

14. John H. Evans, *Playing God? Human Genetic Engineering and the Rationalization of Public Bioethical Debate* (Chicago: University of Chicago Press, 2002).

15. Andrew Pollack, "Engineering by Scientists on Embryo Stirs Criticism," *New York Times*, May 13, 2008, A14.

16. Genetics and Public Policy Center, "Reproductive Genetic Testing: Issues and Options for Policymakers" (Washington, DC, 2004).

17. Charles Taylor, "Liberal Politics and the Public Sphere," in *The New Communitarian Thinking*, ed. Amitai Etzioni (Charlottesville: University Press of Virginia, 1995), 185–86.

18. The studies of powerful institutions in the public sphere generally fall under the headings of social movement theory and social problems theory. In this book, I do not directly engage either of these literatures because I am ultimately not focused on activists. In the social movement literature, the relevant literature is called the "framing literature," which is primarily focused on the actions of elite movement leaders and not the content of the ideas of the potentially mobilized ordinary citizens. According to Oliver and Johnston, "In frame alignment, people's belief systems are taken largely as givens, and movement intellectuals perform the marketing task of packaging their issue so that it will be accepted by others." See Pamela E. Oliver and Hank Johnston, "What a Good Idea! Ideologies and Frames in Social Movement Research," *Mobilization* 4, no. 1 (2000): 47. Something very similar could be said about the social problems literature, which focuses on claims-makers. In the terms of these academic debates, I am examining what Oliver and

Johnston call the "belief systems" of the ordinary citizens that the activists are trying to achieve alignment with or the social problems that advocates are trying to change.

19. John H. Evans and Kathy Hudson, "Religion and Reproductive Genetics: Beyond Views of Embryonic Life?" *Journal for the Scientific Study of Religion* 46, no. 4 (2007): 565–81.

20. Evans, *Playing God? Human Genetic Engineering and the Rationalization of Public Bioethical Debate.*

21. John H. Evans, "Between Technocracy and Democratic Legitimation: A Proposed Compromise Position for Common Morality Public Bioethics," *Journal of Medicine and Philosophy* 31 (2006): 213–34.

22. Arthur Caplan, "'Who Lost China?' A Foreshadowing of Today's Ideological Disputes in Bioethics," *Hastings Center Report* 35, no. 3 (2005): 12–13.

23. Neil Gross and Solon Simmons, "The Religiosity of American College and University Professors," *Sociology of Religion* 70 (2009): 101–29; Elaine Howard Ecklund and Christopher P. Scheitle, "Religion Among Academic Scientists: Distinctions, Disciplines, and Demographics," *Social Problems* 54, no. 2 (2007): 289–307; Elaine Howard Ecklund, *Waging Peace: On the Front Lines of Science and Religion* (New York: Oxford University Press, forthcoming).

24. Ecklund, *Waging Peace: On the Front Lines of Science and Religion.*

25. For example, in an analysis of survey questions on cloning in the United Kingdom, Shepherd and his colleagues break down the religions of the respondents as Church of England, Catholic, other Christian, non-Christian, and none. The first difference with the United States is that nearly half the respondents say "none," whereas about 12 percent of Americans would say "none." Second, although not shown in the paper, the level of adherence by those who retain an identity would be much lower than in the United States. Third, the religious traditions represented are not in synch with the United States. Finally, the very way that religion is used in societal debates in the United Kingdom is different than the United States. For example, the authors speculate that the reason there was "little direct appeal to religion" in their focus groups was that participants had "wariness about explicitly positioning themselves as religious. To have done so may have risked being positioned by others as judgmental, narrow-minded, fundamentalist or in terms of any of the other negative constructions of what it means to be (constructed as) religious within a largely secular cultural context." I think that such negative constructions of religiosity do not exist in general among U.S. citizens. See Richard Shepherd et al., "Towards an Understanding of British Public Attitudes Concerning Human Cloning," *Social Science and Medicine* 65 (2007): 390–91.

26. Celeste M. Condit, "How the Public Understands Genetics: Non-Deterministic and Non-Discriminatory Interpretations of the "Blueprint" Metaphor," *Public Understanding of Science* 8 (1999): 169–80; and Benjamin R. Bates et al., "Warranted Concerns, Warranted Outlooks: A Focus Group Study of Public

Understandings of Genetic Research," *Social Science and Medicine* 60 (2005): 331–44.

27. Social scientists have focused on the experience of the people who use the technologies. See Barbara Katz Rothman, *Recreating Motherhood: Ideology and Technology in a Patriarchal Society* (New York: Norton, 1989); Barbara Katz Rothman, *The Tentative Pregnancy: Prenatal Diagnosis and the Future of Motherhood* (New York: Viking, 1986); Sarah Franklin, *Embodied Progress: A Cultural Account of Assisted Conception* (London and New York: Routledge, 1997); Gay Becker, *The Elusive Embryo: How Women and Men Approach New Reproductive Technologies* (Berkeley and Los Angeles: University of California Press, 2000); and Rayna Rapp, *Testing Women, Testing the Fetus: The Social Impact of Amniocentesis in America* (London and New York: Routledge, 1999). They have also examined the views of those who administer the technologies. See Elizabeth Ettorre, *Reproductive Genetics, Gender and the Body* (London and New York: Routledge, 2002). Scholars have also examined the potential social implications of these technologies, and the nature of elite debates about them. See Troy Duster, *Backdoor to Eugenics* (New York: Routledge, 1990); and Evans, *Playing God? Human Genetic Engineering and the Rationalization of Public Bioethical Debate.* There are many studies of attitudes of particular groups, such as those who have a child with a genetic disorder, adults with a genetic disorder, pregnant women and geneticists. See Dorothy Wertz, S. R. Janes, and R.W. Erbe, "Attitudes Toward the Prenatal Diagnosis of Cystic Fibrosis Factors in Decision-Making Among Affected Families," *American Journal of Human Genetics* 50, no. 5 (1992): 1077–85; L. Henneman et al., "Attitudes Toward Reproductive Issues and Carrier Testing Among Adult Patients and Parents of Children with Cystic Fibrosis (CF)," *Prenatal Diagnosis* 21 (2001): 1–9; Lee A. Learman et al., "Social and Familial Context of Prenatal Genetic Testing Decisions: Are There Racial/Ethnic Differences," *American Journal of Medical Genetics Part C* 119 (2003): 19–26; and Dorothy C. Wertz and John C. Fletcher, *Genetics and Ethics in Global Perspective* (Dordrecht: Kluwer Academic, 2004). These are obviously of limited usefulness for understanding the attitudes of the general public.

28. In the first paper on American attitudes toward prenatal genetic testing, Singer and her colleagues found overwhelmingly favorable attitudes toward prenatal genetic testing with younger people, those with more education and those who follow science news more closely being more supportive. See Eleanor Singer, "Public Attitudes Toward Genetic Testing," *Population Research and Policy Review* 10 (1991): 250. A 1999 study that examined attitudes toward prenatal genetic testing found that women and those with more education think prenatal genetic testing will do more good than harm, and nonwhites and those who attend religious services more often think it will do more harm. See Eleanor Singer, Amy D. Corning, and Toni Antonucci, "Attitudes Toward Genetic Testing and Fetal Diagnosis," *Journal of Health and Social Behavior* 40 (1999): 438. While they did include religious covariates, they found that particular religious affiliation had no effect.

A 2000 study that focuses on attitudes toward prenatal genetic testing also found that church attendance is a significant negative predictor of preferences for testing and that self-identification as Catholic is likewise related to negative altitudes toward testing. See Eleanor Singer, Toni Antonucci, and John Van Hoewyk, "Racial and Ethnic Variations in Knowledge and Attitudes About Genetic Testing," *Genetic Testing* 8, no. 1 (2004): 41. A 1998 paper summarizes opinion change over time in attitudes toward genetic testing, genetic modification and gene therapy using commercial polls, without attempts to determine the variables that predict certain responses. They find little change in awareness or attitudes. See Eleanor Singer, Amy Corning, and Mark Lamias, "The Polls—Trends: Genetic Testing, Engineering and Therapy," *Public Opinion Quarterly* 62 (1998): 635. Bane and her colleagues later engaged in a very similar study, with similar results. See Audra Bane et al., "Life and Death Decisions: America's Changing Attitudes Toward Genetic Engineering, Genetic Testing and Abortion, 1972–98," *International Social Work* 46, no. 2 (2003): 209–19.

Singer's research did not focus on religion, and what we can learn about the views of religious groups can only be determined by looking at her covariates. That said, the sum of this research on attitudes toward reproductive genetic technologies—for our purposes—is simply that attending the services of any religious tradition is associated with greater opposition to reproductive genetic technologies. In a paper with Kathy Hudson that uses the survey data used in this book, I examine how religious tradition determines views of different types of RGTs, but cannot really get at more in-depth questions of why religious people are so opposed. See Evans and Hudson, "Religion and Reproductive Genetics: Beyond Views of Embryonic Life?"

29. Bates et al., "Warranted Concerns, Warranted Outlooks: A Focus Group Study of Public Understandings of Genetic Research"; and Andrea L. Kalfoglou et al., "Opinions About New Reproductive Genetic Technologies: Hopes and Fears for Our Genetic Future," *Fertility and Sterility* 83, no. 6 (2005): 1612–21.

30. Paul DiMaggio and Walter W. Powell, "Introduction," in *The New Institutionalism in Organizational Analysis*, ed. Walter W. Powell and Paul J. DiMaggio (Chicago: University of Chicago Press, 1991), 1–40.

31. I most closely follow Moon in this definition. See Dawne Moon, *God, Sex and Politics: Homosexuality and Everyday Theologies* (Chicago: University of Chicago Press, 2004), 9. Many cultural sociologists use very similar definitions. For example, Swidler writes that discourse is not concerned with "what particular individuals think or believe" but on "how the larger semiotic structure—the discursive possibilities available in a given social world—constrains meaning (by constructing the categories through which people perceive themselves and others or simply by limiting what can be thought and said)." See Ann Swidler, *Talk of Love: How Culture Matters* (Chicago: University of Chicago Press, 2001), 6. Similarly, Eliasoph and Lichterman write that, in current cultural sociology, culture "is

a set of publicly shared codes or repertoires, building blocks that structure people's ability to think and to share ideas. A society's collectively held symbolic system is as binding and real as a language." See Nina Eliasoph and Paul Lichterman, "Culture in Interaction," *American Journal of Sociology* 108, no. 4 (2003): 735.

32. There are obviously many more discourses that could be identified in the data. First, as noted above, I have not focused on the various discourses that are generally used to support RGTs. Second, there are discourses used by opponents that appear less frequently in the data. For parsimony, I do not discuss these further.

33. Bates et al., "Warranted Concerns, Warranted Outlooks: A Focus Group Study of Public Understandings of Genetic Research," 341. See also Rachel Iredale et al., "What Choices Should We Be Able to Make About Designer Babies? A Citizens' Jury of Young People in South Wales," *Health Expectations* 9 (2006): 207–17; Kalfoglou et al., "Opinions About New Reproductive Genetic Technologies: Hopes and Fears for Our Genetic Future.". Survey research also backs this distinction. As Kalfoglou and colleagues note, "Most surveys, including our own . . . , have shown that there is overwhelming public support for the availability of prenatal genetic testing, carrier testing, and new RGTs to avoid disorders like Down syndrome and other conditions that present a serious threat to health . . . . In contrast, these same studies show little support for the hypothetical use of RGTs to select for or alter traits such as intelligence, obesity, or homosexuality." See Kalfoglou et al., "Opinions About New Reproductive Genetic Technologies: Hopes and Fears for Our Genetic Future," 1612–13.

34. For a good summary of theories of healthy debates in the public sphere in relation to the abortion debate, see Myra Marx Ferree et al., *Shaping Abortion Discourse: Democracy and the Public Sphere in German and the United States* (Cambridge and New York: Cambridge University Press, 2002), chap. 10. For Habermas and the deliberative democracy tradition, a good starting point is Amy Gutmann and Dennis Thompson, *Democracy and Disagreement* (Cambridge: Harvard University Press, 1996). For summaries of empirical studies of the purported effects of deliberative democracy, see David M. Ryfe, "Does Deliberative Democracy Work?" *Annual Review of Political Science* 8 (2005): 49–71; Diana C. Mutz, "Is Deliberative Democracy a Falsifiable Theory?" *Annual Review of Political Science* 11, no. 521–38 (2008); and Michael X. Delli Carpini, Fay Lomax Cook, and Lawrence R. Jacobs, "Public Deliberation, Discursive Participation, and Citizen Engagement: A Review of the Empirical Literature," *Annual Review of Political Science* 7 (2004): 315–44.

35. Andrew J. Perrin, "Political Microcultures: Linking Civic Life and Democratic Discourse," *Social Forces* 84, no. 2 (2005): 1049.

36. Diana C. Mutz and Paul S. Martin, "Facilitating Communication Across Lines of Political Difference: The Role of the Mass Media," *American Political Science Review* 95, no. 1 (2001): 97.

37. Examination of the literature on attitude polarization over social issues reveals that it is extremely common for the public to form a common mind about issues over time, presumably through direct or indirect deliberation. See Paul DiMaggio, John Evans, and Bethany Bryson, "Have Americans' Social Attitudes Become More Polarized?" *American Journal of Sociology* 102 (1996): 690–755; John H. Evans, "Have Americans' Attitudes Become More Polarized?—an Update," *Social Science Quarterly* 84, no. 1 (2003): 71–90. For example, whether a Jewish person should be president was a divisive issue for several decades, but now there is near consensus among the public that this is acceptable. We could say the same about interracial marriage, and there also appears to be growing consensus that we as a society should ameliorate global warming. In general, empirical studies of polarization over time show that increasing consensus is the norm and decreasing consensus is more rare, suggesting that actual discussion to reach a common mind does occur.

38. James D. Hunter, *Culture Wars* (New York: Basic, 1991); and Hunter, *Before the Shooting Begins* (New York: Free Press, 1994).

39. DiMaggio, Evans, and Bryson, "Have Americans' Social Attitudes Become More Polarized?"; Evans, "Have Americans' Attitudes Become More Polarized?—an Update."

40. Yonghe Yang and N. J. Demerath III, "What American Culture War? A View from the Trenches as Opposed to the Command Posts and the Press Corps," in *Cultural Wars in American Politics: Critical Reviews of a Popular Thesis*, ed. Rhys H. Williams (Hawthorn: Aldine de Gruyter, 1997); Nancy J. Davis and Robert V. Robinson, "Are Rumors of War Exaggerated? Religious Orthodoxy and Moral Progressivism in America," *American Journal of Sociology* 102, no. 3 (November 1996): 756–76; and John H. Evans, "Worldviews or Social Groups as the Source of Moral Value Attitudes: Implications for the Culture Wars Thesis," *Sociological Forum* 12, no. 3 (1997): 371–404.

41. Morris Fiorina, *Culture War? The Myth of a Polarized America* (New York: Pearson Longman, 2005).

42. DiMaggio, Evans, and Bryson, "Have Americans' Social Attitudes Become More Polarized?"

43. The most clear precursor theory in Hunter is Peter Berger's phenomenology, which was itself a synthesis of many predecessors such as Weber, Schutz, Mead, Durkheim, and others. See Peter L. Berger, *The Sacred Canopy: Elements of a Sociological Theory of Religion* (New York: Doubleday, 1967).

44. DiMaggio, Evans, and Bryson, "Have Americans' Social Attitudes Become More Polarized?"; Evans, "Have Americans' Attitudes Become More Polarized?—an Update."

45. Hunter, *Before the Shooting Begins*, 8–9.

46. Laurence Tribe, *Abortion: The Clash of Absolutes* (New York: Norton, 1992), 27.

47. Simona Goi, "Agonism, Deliberation and the Politics of Abortion," *Polity* 37, no. 1 (2005): 60.

48. David M. Ryfe, "The Practice of Deliberative Democracy: A Study of Sixteen Organizations," *Political Communication* 16 (2002): 376.

49. Robert Huckfeldt, "Unanimity, Discord, and the Communication of Public Opinion," *American Journal of Political Science* 51, no. 4 (2007): 984. See also Diana C. Mutz, "Cross-Cutting Social Networks: Testing Democratic Theory in Practice," *American Political Science Review* 96, no. 1 (2002): 111–26; Mutz and Martin, "Facilitating Communication Across Lines of Political Difference: The Role of the Mass Media."

50. Hunter, *Culture Wars*; Hunter, *Before the Shooting Begins*. In his comprehensive review of the term "ideology" in the social sciences, Gerring concludes that many definitions of ideology are "virtually indistinguishable from worldview, cultural system, symbol-system, or belief-system" in that they are, to use one formulation, "vast receptacle[s] for all conscious and relatively organized ideational phenomena." Gerring concludes that in political science, all definitions of ideology include the idea that ideologies are internally coherent sets of ideas, while the dominant Americanist branch also includes the idea that these are "organized in a hierarchical fashion, in which more specific attitudes interact with attitudes toward the more general class of objects in which the specific object is seen to belong." See John Gerring, "Ideology: A Definitional Analysis," *Political Research Quarterly* 50, no. 4 (1997): 969, 975. For example, Peffley and Hurwitz build on Converse's classic 1964 study to "predict an individual's specific attitudes from a knowledge of the individual's superordinate or abstract attitudes (or vice versa)." To do so they study a " 'hierarchical' model of ideological constraint," a "pyramidal structure . . . organized with more abstract attitudes at the top of the belief system and more specific attitudes subsumed under the general ones." They continue by writing that "the most central elements in the figure are abstract beliefs about the appropriate role of government in different policy domains . . . These beliefs are assumed to constrain more specific preferences for concrete government actions in more defined areas of public policies. . . . Finally, the more general attitudes are assumed to be partially—but not totally—a function of liberalism-conservatism . . . at the apex of the hierarchy." They also "assume that causation flows from the abstract to the specific, so that when an individual is faced with the question of what government should do in a given instance, his or her preference will be based, in part, on more general principles. This model thus assumes a degree of deductive political reasoning, from abstract beliefs to more specific political preferences." See Mark A. Peffley and Jon Hurwitz, "A Hierarchical Model of Attitude Constraint," *American Journal of Political Science* 29 (1985): 872, 876–77. Note that "constraint" and "deductive political reasoning" in this literature refer to what would be called "logic" in the worldview perspective.

Scholars of social movement framing see similarities between ideologies and frames. Oliver and Johnston write that "at a superficial level, ideologies and master frames may seem to be equivalent. Both are broad configurations of ideas within which more specific ideas are included." See Oliver and Johnston, "What a Good Idea! Ideologies and Frames in Social Movement Research," 49. A master frame refers to a more abstract symbolic structure to explain how movements surrounding issues X, Y, and Z are related. See David A. Snow and Robert D. Benford, "Master Frames and Cycles of Protest," in *Frontiers in Social Movement Theory*, ed. Aldon D. Morris and Carol McClurg Mueller (New Haven: Yale University Press, 1992), 133–55. For example, Operation Rescue is a social movement traditionally concerned with blockading abortion clinics to "save unborn babies." Operation Rescue attempted to expand beyond abortion to picket Barnes and Nobles because of some books with naked children in them, and protest at Disney World because of a marketed "gay day" at the theme park.

Why these issues? Youngman follows the activists' accounts by saying that they all flow from the same higher order discursive principle: Reconstructionist theology. "For Reconstructionists, all three of Operation Rescue's protest targets (the clinics, the bookstores, and Disney) represent the ongoing modernization and secularization of American society," she writes. For the activists, these issues were all the same because they are all logically implied by "modernization and secularization." She cites Operation Rescue leaders who saw "strong connections between legalized abortion, Disney's 'homosexual agenda,' and Barnes and Noble's 'child pornography.'" She quotes a leader talking to the press: "It's the same arena, you have to understand . . . We are dealing with two world views, a culture of death vs. a culture of life . . . the homosexual world view is exactly the same as the world view of abortion . . . 'I'll do what I want whenever I want to, and the one commandment I have is "thou shalt not get in my face, and don't you dare judge me!"' . . . It's not a battle about abortion or homosexuality, it's a battle about whose laws reign, or who is Lord, and we're saying that Jesus is Lord and Mickey is not." See Nicole Youngman, "When Frame Extension Fails: Operation Rescue and the 'Triple Gates of Hell' in Orlando," *Journal of Contemporary Ethnography* 32, no. 5 (2003): 529, 535.

While worldview and ideology often connote thought or belief, instead of discourse, framing connotes discourse. However, if we think of what the Operation Rescue leader says above as indicative of their worldview, note that they do articulate these higher, more abstract beliefs as discourses. Finally, the term worldview is ubiquitous in Western intellectual thought. Among the sociological variants, I am de-emphasizing the phenomenological qualities and emphasizing the discursive. Using the closely related concept of "ideology" instead of worldview, my approach follows what Gerring calls the linguistic approach, where "the rules, regularities, and principles of any ideology . . . derive not so much from the intentions of the ideologists (their values and beliefs), but rather from the linguistic norms in which they are embedded." See Gerring, "Ideology: A Definitional Analysis," 967.

51. Hunter, *Culture Wars*, 122.

52. Ibid.

53. Ibid., 127.

54. I demonstrate this empirically in chap. 7.

55. Valerie Jenness, "Social Movement Growth, Domain Expansion, and Framing Processes: The Gay/Lesbian Movement and Violence Against Gays and Lesbians as a Social Problem," *Social Problems* 42, no. 1 (1995): 154. See also Donileen R. Loseke, *Thinking About Social Problems: An Introduction to Constructionist Perspectives* (New York: Aldine de Gruyter, 1999), 82; Joel Best, *Social Problems* (New York: W. W. Norton, 2008), 48. Best says, "Domain expansion and elaboration reflect advocates' preference for inclusive definitions. Many social-problems campaigns begin with activists calling attention to extreme typifying examples in order to mobilize societal consensus. From that narrow foundation, they gradually can extend the problem's domain, arguing that other, less melodramatic cases are another form of, really no different than, the moral equivalent of, or just the same as the original typifying examples, and that the problem is complex, with many facets demanding attention. Such expansive claims help keep the problem visible. Social movements cannot afford to succeed and then relax; once members believe a cause is won, they may drift away. Domain expansion and elaboration let movement leaders argue that the battle continues, that work remains to be done, and that the cause needs continued support. Similarly, extending the domain lets advocates offer the media new angles on a problem, encouraging continued coverage that can keep the problem visible." See Joel Best, *Random Violence: How We Talk About New Crimes and New Victims* (Berkeley and Los Angeles: University of California Press, 1999), 169.

56. Joel Best, *Threatened Children: Rhetoric and Concern About Child-Victims* (Chicago: University of Chicago Press, 1990), chap. 4.

57. "Key Moments in NARAL Pro-Choice America's History": "1993—To more accurately reflect the organization's comprehensive approach to reproductive health policy, NARAL changes its name to the National Abortion and Reproductive Rights Action League" (http://www.prochoiceamerica.org/about-us/learn-about-us/history.html; accessed November 24, 2008). For the Religious Coalition for Reproductive Choice, see http://www.rcrc.org/about/history.cfm (accessed November 24, 2008).

58. Best, *Threatened Children: Rhetoric and Concern About Child-Victims*, chap. 4.

59. Ibid., 68–69.

60. Loseke, *Thinking About Social Problems: An Introduction to Constructionist Perspectives*, 83.

61. Ibid.

62. Youngman, "When Frame Extension Fails: Operation Rescue and the 'Triple Gates of Hell' in Orlando."

63. Richard J. Meagher, "Tax Revolt as a Family Value: How the Christian Right is Becoming a Freemarket Champion," *Public Eye Magazine* 21, no. 1 (2006).

64. By removing the term "embryonic," this term implies something about views of adult life, which it should not. By giving one side the positive prefix "pro"

also implicitly puts them on the moral high ground, while I would like my analysis to be neutral. The term "pro-life" is also conflated with opposition to abortion, and while I will show that that is indeed an obvious empirical association, there are people who oppose abortion without using the embryonic life discourse. Moreover, "non pro-lifer" does not mean that such a person is opposed to "life," only that they do not think that embryonic life should be held to the same esteem as born life. Despite these terminological qualms, the phrases "respondent who uses the embryonic life discourse" and "respondent who does not use the embryonic life discourse" are so cumbersome that they impede understanding, so I decided to use the shorter terms.

65. The social problems literature used here is very similar to examinations of "frame extension" by social movement scholars. See David A. Snow et al., "Frame Alignment Processes, Micromobilization, and Movement Participation," *American Sociological Review* 51 (1986): 464–81; Youngman, "When Frame Extension Fails: Operation Rescue and the 'Triple Gates of Hell' in Orlando." For a sophisticated example of an analysis of how activists changed the discourse used to discuss a social problem, see particularly chaps. 2 and 3 in Joseph E. Davis, *Accounts of Innocence: Sexual Abuse, Trauma, and the Self* (Chicago: University of Chicago Press, 2005).

66. Ethics and Religious Liberty Commission, For Faith and Family Issues, "Sanctity of human life fact sheet – 2004."

67. See http://www.usccb.org/prolife/programs/rlp/Coors05.shtml.

68. Best uses this logic when he shows the percentage of the public that think of different issues as "child sexual abuse." Less successful efforts to make certain situations "child sexual abuse" are indicated by the low percentage of the public who use the discourse "child sexual abuse" to discuss the situation. See Best, *Threatened Children: Rhetoric and Concern About Child-Victims*, 84–85.

69. Here I will follow cognitive psychologists who explain this "fit" or metaphorical similarity as guided by cultural cues in the environment. The cue is some sort of analogy between the situation that the existing discourse has been used previously for and the situation presented to the person. For our purposes, we can use the simple model, which DiMaggio explains using the cognitive psychology term for discourse of "schemata." (There are obviously differences in the technical meanings of the terms discourse and schemata, but for my limited purposes I can treat them as analogous.) The cue is made where "two schemata or related structures lend themselves to analogy (and thus to generalization across domains) insofar as they share particular features . . . that create a correspondence between them." See Paul DiMaggio, "Culture and Cognition," *Annual Review of Sociology* 23 (1997): 274, 281. For example, people rely on visual and physical cues when invoking schema having to do with persons. The "welfare mother" schema is activated by the stereotypical appearance of such a person. See Susan T. Fiske and Shelley E. Taylor, *Social Cognition* (New York: McGraw-Hill, 1991), 144.

70. Karen A. Cerulo, *Culture in Mind: Toward a Sociology of Culture and Cognition* (New York: Routledge, 2002), 58–60.

71. Carl Hulse, "Democrats Weigh Methods for Ending Stem Cell Ban," *New York Times*, March 1, 2009, A:11.

72. Erik Parens and Lori P. Knowles, "Reprogenetics and Public Policy: Reflections and Recommendations," *Hastings Center Report* 33, no. 4 (2003): S10.

73. Hanna et al. in Ruth Ellen Bulger, Elizabeth Meyer Bobby, and Harvey V. Fineberg, *Society's Choices: Social and Ethical Decision Making in Biomedicine* (Washington, DC: National Academy Press, 1995), 187.

74. Hunter, *Before the Shooting Begins*, 8.

75. Smith shows that worldviews are more compatible than the worldview imagery suggests. See Christian Smith, *American Evangelicalism: Embattled and Thriving* (Chicago: University of Chicago Press, 1998), 104–7. Even Peter Berger, one of the architects of the notion that the presence of two worldviews in the same interactive space will lead to the delegitimation of both, has come to the conclusion that this presumption was a mistake. See Peter L. Berger, "The Desecularization of the World: A Global Overview," in *The Desecularization of the World: Resurgent Religion and World Politics*, ed. Peter L. Berger (Grand Rapids: Eerdmans, 1999), 1–18. Moreover, many recent innovations in cultural sociology have concluded that we actually know much more culture than we regularly use, including, presumably, discourses that would logically be opposed to other discourses that the worldview perspective would place in separate worldviews. See DiMaggio, "Culture and Cognition"; Swidler, *Talk of Love: How Culture Matters*. Studies also show that the highest-level discursive elements in worldviews are very weak predictors of attitudes on social issues, suggesting the structure needs to be loosened to allow in additional factors. See Evans, "Worldviews or Social Groups as the Source of Moral Value Attitudes: Implications for the Culture Wars Thesis." Political scientists have also long known that ordinary people are not coherent in their attitudes. See Gerring, "Ideology: A Definitional Analysis."

76. Swidler, *Talk of Love: How Culture Matters*, 182. If the cultural systems approaches, such as the worldview idea, have too much structure, Swidler's original model of culture as a "tool kit" has been described as structureless. See Ilana Friedrich Silber, "Pragmatic Sociology as Cultural Sociology: Beyond Repertoire Theory?" *European Journal of Social Theory* 6, no. 4 (2003): 431; Ann Swidler, "Culture in Action: Symbols and Strategies," *American Sociological Review* 51 (1986): 273–86. Swidler's 2001 book-length statement adds some structure. Silber has concluded that only what she calls French "pragmatic sociology" has attempted "to introduce some form of order or structure in cultural 'tool-kits' or repertoires that other repertoire theorists have tended to leave largely unstructured or to structure in much rougher, less detailed fashion." See Silber, "Pragmatic Sociology as Cultural Sociology: Beyond Repertoire Theory?" 435. In the words of William Sewell, Jr., "Our job as cultural analysts is to discern what the shapes and consistencies of local meanings actually are and to determine how, why, and to what extent they hang together." See William H. Sewell, Jr., "The Concept(s) of Culture,"

in *Beyond the Cultural Turn: New Directions in the Study of Society and Culture*, ed. Victoria E. Bonnell and Lynn Hunt (Berkeley: University of California Press, 1999), 58.

77. Michele Dillon, "The American Abortion Debate: Culture War or Normal Discourse?" in *The American Culture Wars: Current Contests and Future Prospects*, ed. James L. Nolan (Charlottesville: University Press of Virginia, 1996), 117.

78. Dillon, "The American Abortion Debate: Culture War or Normal Discourse?" 119.

79. This presumes that people on both sides of the abortion divide have not socially selected their interaction networks so as to never encounter someone who has opposing views. A network study of deliberation about controversial topics in communication networks suggests that this is not the case as people in the same network do have discordant views about abortion, even if they try to avoid talking about abortion. See Huckfeldt, "Unanimity, Discord, and the Communication of Public Opinion."

80. In fig. 3, I represent opposition and support for types of abortion other than abortion for fetal defect. This is only done to connect my argument to claims in the culture wars thesis, because I did not ask the respondents about these other types of abortion. Hunter's thesis presumes—fairly reasonably—that people who are opposed to all or most types of abortion would use this discourse.

81. Cystic Fibrosis Foundation, "About Cystic Fibrosis" (http://www.cff.org/AboutCF/; accessed May 14, 2008).

82. Peter J. Thuesen, "The Logic of Mainline Churchliness: Historical Background Since the Reformation," in *The Quiet Hand of God: Faith-Based Activism and the Public Role of Mainline Protestantism*, ed. Robert Wuthnow and John H. Evans (Berkeley: University of California Press, 2002), 27–53.

83. Robert Wuthnow and John H. Evans, *The Quiet Hand of God: Faith-Based Activism and the Public Role of Mainline Protestantism* (Berkeley: University of California Press, 2002).

84. Wuthnow and Evans, *The Quiet Hand of God: Faith-Based Activism and the Public Role of Mainline Protestantism*, 4.

85. Robert D. Woodberry and Christian S. Smith, "Fundamentalism et al: Conservative Protestants in America," *Annual Review of Sociology* 24 (1998): 25–56.

86. Donald E. Miller, *Reinventing American Protestantism: Christianity in the New Millennium* (Berkeley and Los Angeles: University of California Press, 1997); and Kimon Howland Sargeant, *Seeker Churches: Promoting Traditional Religion in a Nontraditional Way* (New Brunswick: Rutgers University Press, 2000).

87. Smith, *American Evangelicalism: Embattled and Thriving*.

88. For a particularly influential categorization of survey respondents into these Protestant categories by denomination, see Brian Steensland et al., "The Measure of American Religion: Toward Improving the State of the Art," *Social Forces* 79, no. 1 (2000): 291–318.

89. With the members of congregations, I struggled with whether to interview a random sample of people who were members of congregations or to interview those who might be more aware of the discourse used in their tradition. In the end, half the interviews were conducted with a random sample of members from religious congregations, and half from those considered by the religious leader of the congregation to be able to "do a good job in discussing this issue." Therefore, my interviews represent something between these two categories. These people were by no means religious experts. They were truly ordinary members, with those identified as being "good at talking about this issue" being slightly more articulate. Examination of the conclusions about these technologies reached by the two types of members suggests they are broadly similar in their views.

Chapter Two

1. There have been a few attempts to evaluate ordinary religious persons' views historically, primarily of the eugenics movement. See Christine Rosen, *Preaching Eugenics: Religious Leaders and the American Eugenics Movement* (New York: Oxford University Press, 2004); Amy Laura Hall, *Conceiving Parenthood: American Protestantism and the Spirit of Reproduction* (Grand Rapids: Eerdmans, 2008).

2. Thomas F. Lee, *The Human Genome Project: Cracking the Genetic Code of Life* (New York: Plenum Press, 1991), 38.

3. Ibid., 31.

4. Ibid., 35.

5. Daniel Kevles, *In the Name of Eugenics: Genetics and the Uses of Human Heredity* (Berkeley and Los Angeles: University of California Press, 1985), ix. My description of the nineteenth-century eugenics movement is based on the canonical texts by Kevles and Paul. See Diane B. Paul, *Controlling Human Heredity: 1865 to the Present* (Amherst: Humanity Books, 1995).

6. Kevles, *In the Name of Eugenics: Genetics and the Uses of Human Heredity*, 34.

7. Ibid., 44, 47.

8. Ibid., 47.

9. Ibid., 97.

10. Ibid., 164.

11. Ibid., 118.

12. Ibid., 110–11.

13. Rosen, *Preaching Eugenics: Religious Leaders and the American Eugenics Movement*.

14. Ibid., chap. 5.

15. Ibid.

16. Hermann J. Muller, "The Guidance of Human Evolution," *Perspectives in Biology and Medicine* 3, no. 1 (1959): 15.

17. Evans, *Playing God? Human Genetic Engineering and the Rationalization of Public Bioethical Debate*, 53–56.

18. John Fletcher, "The Brink: The Parent-Child Bond in the Genetic Revolution," *Theological Studies* 33, no. 3 (1972): 484.

19. Rebecca Rae Anderson, *Religious Traditions and Prenatal Genetic Counseling* (Omaha: Munroe-Meyer Institute, Univ. of Nebraska Medical Center, 2002).

20. Tracy M. Sonneborn, *The Control of Human Heredity and Evolution* (New York: Macmillan, 1965).

21. Hermann J. Muller, "Means and Aims in Human Betterment," in *The Control of Human Heredity and Evolution*, ed. T. M. Sonneborn (New York: Macmillan, 1965), 100–22.

22. Julian Huxley, "Eugenics in Evolutionary Perspective," *Perspectives in Biology and Medicine* Winter (1963):173.

23. Evans, *Playing God? Human Genetic Engineering and the Rationalization of Public Bioethical Debate*.

24. By the 1980s, the first experiments with this technology began, but a recent summary concludes that this has yet to be proven an effective treatment for genetic disease (http://www.ornl.gov/sci/techresources/Human_Genome/medicine/genetherapy.shtml).

25. Evans, *Playing God? Human Genetic Engineering and the Rationalization of Public Bioethical Debate*, chap. 4.

26. Ibid., 168–69.

27. Ronald Cole-Turner, "Religion and the Question of Human Germline Modification," in *Design and Destiny: Jewish and Christian Perspectives on Human Germline Modification*, ed. Ronald Cole-Turner (Cambridge: MIT Press, 2008), 1–27.

28. Evans, *Playing God? Human Genetic Engineering and the Rationalization of Public Bioethical Debate*, 168–69; and Cole-Turner, "Religion and the Question of Human Germline Modification," 10.

29. Cole-Turner, "Religion and the Question of Human Germline Modification."

30. Nigel M. de S. Cameron and Amy Michelle DeBaets, "Germline Gene Modification and the Human Condition Before God," in *Design and Destiny*, 93–118.

31. For an account of how this legal situation developed, see James C. Mohr, *Abortion in America: The Origins and Evolution of National Policy* (New York: Oxford University Press, 1978).

32. David J. Garrow, *Liberty and Sexuality: The Right to Privacy and the Making of Roe v. Wade* (New York: Macmillan/Lisa Drew, 1994), 277.

33. Garrow, *Liberty and Sexuality: The Right to Privacy and the Making of Roe v. Wade*, 285–91.

34. John H. Evans, "Multi-Organizational Fields and Social Movement Organization Frame Content: The Religious Pro-Choice Movement," *Sociological Inquiry* 67, no. 4 (1997): 451–69.

35. J. Gordon Melton, *The Churches Speak On: Abortion* (Detroit: Gale Research, 1989), 162.

36. Ibid., 153.

37. Arlene Carmen and Howard Moody, *Abortion Counseling and Social Change From Illegal Act to Medical Practice: The Story of the Clergy Consultation Service on Abortion* (Valley Forge: Judson Press, 1973); Garrow, *Liberty and Sexuality*; and Tom Davis, *Sacred Work: Planned Parenthood and Its Clergy Alliances* (New Brunswick: Rutgers University Press, 2005).

38. Kristin Luker, *Abortion and the Politics of Motherhood* (Berkeley and Los Angeles: University of California Press, 1984).

39. Melton, *Churches Speak On: Abortion*, 163.

40. Evans, "Multi-Organizational Fields and Social Movement Organization Frame Content: The Religious Pro-Choice Movement."

41. Ibid.

42. Melton, *Churches Speak On: Abortion*.

43. Ted G. Jelen and Clyde Wilcox, "Causes and Consequences of Public Attitudes Toward Abortion: A Review and Research Agenda," *Political Research Quarterly* 56, no. 4 (2003): 494.

44. Robert C. Liebman and Robert Wuthnow, eds., *The New Christian Right* (New York: Aldine, 1983).

45. Jelen and Wilcox, "Causes and Consequences of Public Attitudes Toward Abortion: A Review and Research Agenda," 494.

46. John H. Evans, "Polarization in Abortion Attitudes in U.S. Religious Traditions 1972–1998," *Sociological Forum* 17, no. 3 (2002): 397–422.

47. R. G. Edwards and Ruth E. Fowler, "Human Embryos in the Laboratory," *Scientific American* 223, no. 6 (1970): 54.

48. Bentley Glass, *Science and Ethical Values* (Chapel Hill: University of North Carolina Press, 1965), 61.

49. In this passage, homologous means between married couples. See "Instruction on Respect for Human Life in its Origin and on the Dignity of Procreation: Replies to Certain Questions of the Day" (http://www.vatican.va/roman_curia/congregations/cfaith).

50. Tony Reichhardt, "Studies of Faith," *Nature* 432 (2004): 668.

51. *Christian Telegraph*, "Albert Mohler: All involved with IVF responsible for 'human tragedy'" (http://www.christiantelegraph.com/issue319.html).

52. Ivar Bleiklie, Malcolm L. Goggin, and Christine Rothmayr, *Comparative Biomedical Policy: Governing Assisted Reproductive Technologies* (London and New York: Routledge, 2004), 229–30.

53. A. H. Handyside et al., "Pregnancies from Biopsied Human Preimplantation Embryos Sexed by Y-Specific DNA Amplification," *Nature* 344 (1990): 768–70.

54. On preimplantation genetic diagnosis, see Y. Verlinsky et al., "Preimplantation Diagnosis for Early-Onset Alzheimer Disease Caused by V717L Mutation," *JAMA* 287, no. 8 (2002): 1018–21. On preimplantation genetic diagnosis for sex, see http://www.fertility-docs.com/fertility_gender.phtml.

55. See, for example, "Shall we clone a man?" in Paul Ramsey, *Fabricated Man: The Ethics of Genetic Control* (New Haven: Yale University Press, 1970), 60–103.

56. David M. Rorvik, *In His Image: The Cloning of a Man* (Philadelphia: Lippincott, 1978).

57. Kolata, Gina, "Scientists Use Monkey Clones for Stem Cells," *New York Times*, November 15, 2007, A1.

58. John H. Evans, "Religion and Human Cloning: An Exploratory Analysis of the First Available Opinion Data," *Journal for the Scientific Study of Religion* 41, no. 4 (2002): 747–58.

59. There are questions about three technologies (preimplantation genetic diagnosis, human genetic engineering, and amniocentesis) for each of five purposes (to avoid a fatal childhood disease, to avoid adult onset disease, to select for intelligence or strength in offspring, or to determine sex) and a question about reproductive cloning. The respondent is told what each technology entails before being asked the question. They are told that amniocentesis ("prenatal genetic testing") is "genetic testing that is done during pregnancy to find out if the fetus has or is likely to develop certain inherited diseases or characteristics. Test results may be used to help parents prepare for the birth of that child or make a decision about terminating the pregnancy." They are told of preimplantation genetic diagnosis that it is "genetic testing that is done on embryos produced through in vitro fertilization before they are transferred to a woman's womb. Based on the test results, parents can select which embryos to transfer into the woman's womb. For example, they may want to select only embryos with no genetic diseases, those of a specific sex, or those that have other characteristics. Left over embryos may be discarded, frozen and stored for future use, donated to other couples, or used for research." They are told that genetic modification is "a technique to change the DNA or genes of a person in order to produce particular inherited characteristics." Finally, cloning is "the process of making a genetic copy of an animal or a human from a single cell." Respondents are asked if they strongly approve, approve, disapprove, or strongly disapprove in each instance.

Chapter Three

1. Public opinion studies show that the embryonic life discourse is the primary discourse used to oppose abortion. For example, a study of abortion discourse in the U.S. media found that fetal life was the most prominent antiabortion argument and that the individual rights argument is the most prominent of the pro-choice arguments. See Ferree et al., *Shaping Abortion Discourse: Democracy and the Public*

Sphere in German and the United States, 117–19. In their review of research on attitudes towards abortion, Jelen and Wilcox conclude that research on abortion has revealed that "a number of basic orientations . . . are strong predictors of abortion attitudes. . . . One such general attitudinal gestalt is, of course, respect for human life. Conceptually, the connection between the general value one places on human life and one's attitude about legal abortion seems virtually self-evident." See Jelen and Wilcox, "Causes and Consequences of Public Attitudes Toward Abortion: A Review and Research Agenda," 493.

2. Michele Dillon, "Argumentative Complexity of Abortion Discourse," *Public Opinion Quarterly* 57 (1993): 312. It has also been found that the integrative complexity of the Catholic Church's discourse about abortion in various forums and across time is "relatively low." See also Michele Dillon, "Institutional Legitimation and Abortion: Monitoring the Catholic Church's Discourse," *Journal for the Scientific Study of Religion* 34, no. 2 (1995): 148.

3. Dillon, "Argumentative Complexity of Abortion Discourse," 312.

4. Dillon, "Institutional Legitimation and Abortion: Monitoring the Catholic Church's Discourse," 141, 142.

5. Jennifer Strickler and Nicholas L. Danigelis, "Changing Frameworks in Attitudes Toward Abortion," *Sociological Forum* 17, no. 2 (2002): 199.

6. "Keynote speech," Conference on Genetic and Reproductive Ethics: The Scientific Cutting Edge and the Everyday Healthcare Challenges, Center for Bioethics and Human Dignity (Chicago), July 2005.

7. Leon Kass, "Defending Human Dignity," in *Human Dignity and Bioethics* (Washington, DC: President's Council on Bioethics, 2008), 305.

8. Nigel M. De S. Cameron, "The Prolife Cause and the Coming Revolution: Abortion and the Death of Man," Center for Bioethics and Human Dignity, (http://www.personhood.net/strategy/strategy).

9. In the conclusion, I will address how the inevitable selection of the order of questions influences the breadth of my conclusions.

10. Details obscured to protect anonymity.

11. The survey asked respondents to rank the moral worth of a number of entities, from sperm to advanced fetuses. Those who ascribed "maximum moral worth" to a "human embryo in a woman's womb" (45 percent of the overall sample) were considered to have one marker of using the embryonic life discourse. The survey also asked "what statement best describes your thoughts on the beginning of life?" The choices were various points from "life begins before a sperm fertilizes an egg" to "life begins at birth." Those who selected "life begins when a sperm fertilizes an egg," by far the largest response category, were also considered to have a marker indicating they use the embryonic life discourse. Those who had both markers were considered to be using embryonic life discourse.

The survey also asked the following: "In general, do you agree of disagree with the following statements: suffering is part of what makes us human"; "In general, do you agree of disagree with the following statements: only God should change the genes of the human species"; and "Suppose that genetic testing, genetic modification, and cloning become widespread, on a scale from one to four, how concerned would you be about the following: increased discrimination against the disabled." I take these as indicators of the meaningful suffering, Promethean fatalism, and individual dignity/equality discourses, respectively.

12. As we can see from table 2, the strongest opponents are those opposed to both health and enhancement applications of RGTs. This is also what I find among the qualitative interviews in subsequent chapters. Therefore, I combined the responses to the prenatal testing, preimplantation genetic diagnosis and human genetic engineering survey questions that asked about using these technologies for health applications: avoiding a fatal childhood disease and avoiding an adult onset disease. From these I created a "health applications" index. I created a similar "enhancement" applications index by combining the responses to the questions about using each technology to determine gender and intelligence or strength, as well as reproductive cloning. Limiting the sample to frequent attenders of religious services—so as to match the qualitative data—I split each of these indices at the median into strong and weak opponents of health or enhancement applications. To match the qualitative analysis in later chapters, I consider strong opponents of RGTs in the survey to be those who are strong opponents of both heath and enhancement applications, and weak opponents of RGTs to be those who are strong opponents of enhancements but weak opponents of health applications.

13. An additive index of all the RGT questions shown in table 2 (Chronbach alpha = .94) was correlated with the Promethean fatalism, dignity/equality, and meaningful suffering variables. The coefficients were .31, .10, and .13, respectively, and all are significant at the $p < .001$ level.

Chapter Four

1. James Boyle, "How to give natures a chance," *Times Literary Supplement* July 24, 1998, 21.

2. Becker, *The Elusive Embryo: How Women and Men Approach New Reproductive Technologies*, 6–7.

3. Lorraine Daston and Fernando Vidal, *The Moral Authority of Nature* (Chicago: University of Chicago Press, 2004), 2.

4. Francis Fukuyama argues that "the idea that human rights can be based on human nature has been vigorously attacked from the eighteenth century to the present." Like others, Fukuyama says the attack starts with Hume, moving through twentieth-century analytic philosophy, the same analytic philosophy that gave birth to bioethics. See Fukuyama, *Our Posthuman Future: Consequences of the Biotechnology Revolution*, 112.

5. Latin for "the war of all against all."

6. Cited in Daston and Vidal, *Moral Authority of Nature*, 2.

7. Kate Soper, *What is Nature? Culture, Politics, and the Non-Human* (Cambridge: Blackwell, 1995), 7.

8. Mary Douglas, *How Institutions Think* (Syracuse: Syracuse University Press, 1986).

9. John H. Haldane, "Natural Law and Ethical Pluralism," in *The Many and the One*, ed. Richard Madsen and Tracy B. Strong (Princeton: Princeton University Press, 2003), 90.

10. Haldane, "Natural Law and Ethical Pluralism," 93–94.

11. Caplan, " 'Who Lost China?' A Foreshadowing of Today's Ideological Disputes in Bioethics." I would argue that what has actually happened is that the latter intellectual group retreated from bioethical debate in the 1970s and the 1980s, and returned to power at the hands of a Republican administration that supported their views.

12. Arnhart argues, in general, that "Much of conservative social thought has been devoted to supporting the natural law tradition of Aristotle, Aquinas, and Hume as an alternative to the cultural relativism of Hobbes, Marx and Freud." See Larry Arnhart, "Darwinian Conservatism as the New Natural Law," *Good Society* 12, no. 3 (2003): 16.

13. Fukuyama, *Our Posthuman Future: Consequences of the Biotechnology Revolution*, 112.

14. Ibid., 139.

15. Ibid., 130. Another bioethicist who is often placed in the neoconservative category, Leon Kass, says that cloning "is a radical departure from the natural human way, confounding all normal understandings of father, mother, sibling, grandparent, etc." See Leon R. Kass, "The Wisdom of Repugnance," *The New Republic*, 2/June (1997): 21. Conservative James Q. Wilson thinks that in our assessment of biotechnology we must "ultimately appeal to our natural moral sentiments and natural desires as rooted in our human biological nature." See Arnhart, "Darwinian Conservatism as the New Natural Law," 18. Critics from the left-liberal group tend to call these thinkers "neo-Aristotelian," to signify their connection to the ancient natural law tradition, and not to the Catholic natural law tradition.

16. Ted Peters, *Playing God? Genetic Determinism and Human Freedom* (New York: Routledge, 2003).

17. Patrick D. Hopkins, "Protecting God from Science and Technology: How Religious Criticisms of Biotechnologies Backfire," *Zygon* 37, no. 2 (2002): 317–43.

18. Ibid., 319.

19. Ibid., 320–21.

20. Ibid., 321–22.

21. Ibid., 324.

22. Ibid., 322–24.

23. Ibid., 327.

24. Allen Verhey, " 'Playing God' and Invoking a Perspective," *Journal of Medicine and Philosophy* 20 (1995): 347–64.

25. Hopkins, "Protecting God from Science and Technology: How Religious Criticisms of Biotechnologies Backfire," 339.

26. This definition is inspired by one used in the health effects of religious fatalism literature. See Monica D. Franklin, David G. Schlundt, and Kenneth A. Wallston, "Development and Validation of a Religious Health Fatalism Measure for the African American Faith Community," *Journal of Health Psychology* 13, no. 3 (2008): 324.

27. Ibid., 324.

28. Joseph Fletcher, "Ethical Aspects of Genetic Controls," *New England Journal of Medicine* 285, no. 14 (1971): 781.

29. James D. Watson, "Why Darwin's Still a Scientific Hotshot," *Los Angeles Times Calendar Live*, September 18, 2005.

30. Lee M. Silver, "Reprogenetics: How Reproductive and Genetic Technologies Will Be Combined to Provide New Opportunities for People to Reach Their Reproductive Goals," in *Engineering the Human Germline*, ed. Gregory Stock and John Campbell (New York: Oxford University Press, 2000), 57–71.

31. John Harris, *Clones, Genes and Immortality: Ethics and the Genetic Revolution* (New York: Oxford University Press, 1998), 177–78.

32. Evans, *Playing God? Human Genetic Engineering and the Rationalization of Public Bioethical Debate*, 125.

33. Harris, *Clones, Genes and Immortality: Ethics and the Genetic Revolution*, 177–78.

34. Gregory E. Pence, *Who's Afraid of Human Cloning?* (Lanham: Rowman and Littlefield, 1998), 119.

35. Pence, *Who's Afraid of Human Cloning?* 122.

36. http://www.tvacres.com/advertising_mascots.htm.

37. Haldane, "Natural Law and Ethical Pluralism," 94.

38. The survey asks, "In general, do you agree of disagree with the following statements: Only God should change the genes of the human species." The response ranges from one to four as follows: "1" is "strongly agree," "2" is "agree," "3" is "disagree," and "4" is "strongly disagree." The correlation coefficient between the overall RGT index described in endnote 13 of chap. 3 and this variable is $-.3050$ ($p < .001$)

39. Generalizations created to protect anonymity of respondent.

40. Details obscured to protect anonymity.

41. Details obscured to protect anonymity.

42. Details obscured to protect anonymity.

43. See endnotes 11 and 12 in chap. 3 for a description of how pro-lifers and non–pro-lifers, as well as opponents and proponents, were demarcated using the survey.

44. I ran an ordered logistic regression model with the four-response Promethean fatalism question as the dependent variable, where lower numbers indicate more agreement with the Promethean fatalist discourse, and dummy variables representing high attenders in the various religious traditions as the independent variables. A dummy variable containing all low attenders was the reference group. All coefficients were significant at the $p < .001$ level except the liberal Catholic coefficient, which was significant at the $p < .05$ level. The coefficients are as follows: Fundamentalist Protestant, -1.46; Evangelical Protestant, -1.85; Mainline Protestant, -0.910; Liberal Protestant, -0.582; Traditionalist Catholic, -1.43; Moderate Catholic, -0.886; Liberal Catholic, -0.417; and Other Attender, -1.14.

45. Transubstantiation is where the bread and the wine become the literal body and blood of Christ during the Eucharist ritual.

46. For a classic discussion of this distinction, see Guy E. Swanson, *Religion and Regime: A Sociological Account of the Reformation* (Ann Arbor: University of Michigan Press, 1967). For a useful, short discussion, see Marsha Witten, *All is Forgiven: The Secular Message in American Protestantism* (Princeton: Princeton University Press, 1993), 32–34.

47. http://www.crossroadsinitiative.com/library_article/634/God___The_Father.html.

48. Description of Hunter study by Witten, *All is Forgiven: The Secular Message in American Protestantism*, 34. Hunter's original study is in James Hunter, *American Evangelicalism: Conservative Religion and the Quandary of Modernity* (New Brunswick: Rutgers University Press, 1983), 73–101.

Chapter Five

1. C. S. Lewis, *The Screwtape Letters*, 1943, p. 92. The idea for using this quote came from Mary M. Keys, "Personal Dignity and the Common Good: A Twentieth-Century Thomistic Dialogue," in *Catholicism, Liberalism, and Communitarianism: The Catholic Intellectual Tradition and the Moral Foundations of Democracy*, ed. Kenneth L. Grasso, Gerard V. Bradley and Robert P. Hunt (Lanham: Rowman and Littlefield, 1995), 173.

2. Ruth Macklin, "Dignity is a Useless Concept," *BMJ* 327 (2003): 1419–20; Richard E. Ashcroft, "Making Sense of Dignity," *Journal of Medical Ethics* 31 (2005): 679–82; Timothy Caulfield and Roger Brownsword, "Human Dignity: A Guide to Policy Making in the Biotechnology Era?" *Nature Reviews Genetics* 7 (2006): 72–76; and President's Council on Bioethics, *Human Dignity and Bioethics* (Washington, DC: President's Council on Bioethics, 2008).

3. Macklin, "Dignity is a Useless Concept."

4. President's Council on Bioethics, *Human Cloning and Human Dignity: An Ethical Inquiry* (Washington, DC: President's Council on Bioethics, 2002); President's Council on Bioethics, *Human Dignity and Bioethics.*

5. Daryl Pullman, "Universalism, Particularism and the Ethics of Dignity," *Christian Bioethics* 7, no. 3 (2001): 337; David Gelernter, "The Irreducibly Religious Character of Human Dignity," in *Human Dignity and Bioethics* (Washington, DC: President's Council on Bioethics, 2008), 387–405.

6. Pullman, "Universalism, Particularism and the Ethics of Dignity," 341. There are other meanings of dignity used in bioethics. For extensive discussion of these meanings, see President's Council on Bioethics, *Human Dignity and Bioethics.*

7. Pullman, "Universalism, Particularism and the Ethics of Dignity," 352–53.

8. Eric Cohen, "Of Embryos and Empire," *New Atlantis* 2 (2003): 7–8.

9. Gilbert Meilaender, "Designing Our Descendants," *First Things* 109 (January 2001): 25–28.

10. In the survey, I have a measure of concern with class stratification. The survey asked the following: "Suppose that genetic testing, genetic modification, and cloning became widespread. On a scale from one to four, how concerned would you be about the following: Some people being unable to afford the technology" ("1" is "very concerned" and "4" is "not at all concerned"). The correlation coefficient between the overall RGT index described in chap. 2 (higher numbers mean more opposition) and this variable is .1614 ($p < .001$). That is, those who use this discourse are *less* opposed to RGTs than those who do not use this discourse.

11. There is a correlation of −.10 ($p < .001$) between the RGT index described above in endnote 13 in chap. 3 and the question, "Suppose that genetic testing, genetic modification, and cloning became widespread. On a scale from 1 to 4, how concerned would you be about the following: increased discrimination against the disabled." While I would have preferred to have a greater range of questions that measured use of individual dignity/equality discourses, this question taps discrimination, which is treating an individual person differently because of his or her characteristics. It is different from the concern with setting up a society based on people's characteristics, which is the hallmark of the social dignity/equality discourse.

12. Details obscured to protect anonymity.

13. Details obscured to protect anonymity.

14. See endnotes 11 and 12 in chap. 3 for a description of how pro-lifers and non–pro-lifers, as well as opponents and proponents, were demarcated using the survey.

15. An ordered logistic regression model was run with the four-response individual equality question (described above in endnote 11) as the dependent variable, where lower numbers indicate more agreement with the individual dignity/equality discourse, and dummy variables representing high attenders in the various

religious traditions as the independent variables. Low attenders are the reference group. All coefficients were significant at the $p < .05$ level, except for the mainline Protestant and traditionalist Catholic coefficients, which are not statistically different from the reference group. The coefficients are as follows: Fundamentalist Protestant, –.365; Evangelical Protestant, –.588; Mainline Protestant, –.237; Liberal Protestant, –.363; Traditionalist Catholic, –.266; Moderate Catholic, –.296; Liberal Catholic, –.789; and Other Attender, –.189.

16. Galatians 3:28 (New Revised Standard Version).

17. Hugh Heclo, *Christianity and American Democracy* (Cambridge: Harvard University Press, 2007), 48.

18. An ordered logistic regression model was run with the four-response social equality question (described above in endnote 10) as the dependent variable, where lower numbers indicate more agreement with the social dignity/equality discourse, and dummy variables representing high attenders in the various religious traditions as the independent variables. Low attenders are the reference group. Only the coefficients for the fundamentalist Protestants and evangelical Protestants were significant at .05 and .001, respectively. The coefficients are as follows: Fundamentalist Protestant, .353; Evangelical Protestant, .521; Mainline Protestant, –.064; Liberal Protestant, –.237; Traditionalist Catholic, .305; Moderate Catholic, –.072; Liberal Catholic, –.431; and Other Attender, .179.

19. Andrew Greeley, *The Catholic Imagination* (Berkeley and Los Angeles: University of California Press, 2000), 128.

20. Emile Durkheim, *Suicide* (New York: Free Press, 1951).

21. Quoted in Greeley, *The Catholic Imagination*, 124.

22. To take but one example of official concern with social justice derived from this more social view, in the 1971 statement of the World Synod of Catholic Bishops titled "Justice in the World," the synod wrote: "Listening to the cry of those who suffer violence and are oppressed by unjust systems and structures, and hearing the appeal of a world that by its perversity contradicts the plan of its Creator, we have shared our awareness of the Church's vocation to be present in the heart of the world by proclaiming the Good News to the poor, freedom to the oppressed, and joy to the afflicted." These statements can be found in the Catholic social teaching section Web site of the office for social justice of the Archdiocese of St. Paul and Minneapolis (http://www.osjspm.org/catholic_social_teaching .aspx).

23. Andrew Greeley, "Protestant and Catholic: Is the Analogical Imagination Extinct?" *American Sociological Review* 54 (1989): 486.

24. Greeley, "Protestant and Catholic: Is the Analogical Imagination Extinct?"; Greeley, *The Catholic Imagination*.

25. For a good summary of the Social Gospel movement, see chapter 47 of Sydney Ahlstrom's canonical work, *A Religious History of the American People* (New Haven: Yale University Press, 1972).

26. Michael O. Emerson and Christian Smith, *Divided by Faith: Evangelical Religion and the Problem of Race* (New York: Oxford University Press, 2000).

Chapter Six

1. Quoted in "Infertility/Reproductive Tech Standards 4 Life," Christian Medical and Dental Association (http://www.cmdahome.org).

2. A focus group based study of the general public's view of RGTs has found that there were major disagreements among respondents about the meaning of suffering. See Andrea L. Kalfoglou et al., "Opinions About New Reproductive Genetic Technologies: Hopes and Fears for Our Genetic Future," *Fertility and Sterility* 83, no. 6 (2005): 1612–21. Although the authors of the study do not explicitly link each view to conclusions about RGTs, differing views of suffering was a major distinction in public discourse about the issue.

3. On the history of progress in Western civilization, see Robert Nisbet, *History of the Idea of Progress* (New Brunswick: Transaction Press, 1994).

4. I think I heard this from Stanley Hauerwas at a conference presentation. I do not know whether this observation is original to him.

5. Eric J. Cassell, *The Nature of Suffering and the Goals of Medicine* (New York: Oxford University Press, 1991), 33.

6. David E. Boeyink, "Pain and Suffering," *Journal of Religious Ethics* 2 (1974): 85–98; David H. Smith, "Suffering, Medicine, and Christian Theology," in *On Moral Medicine: Theological Perspectives in Medical Ethics*, ed. Stephen E. Lammers and Allen Verhey (Grand Rapids: Eerdmans, 1987), 255–61; Warren Thomas Reich, "Speaking of Suffering: A Moral Account of Compassion," *Soundings* 72, no. 1 (1989): 83–108; and Courtney S. Campbell, "The Ordeal and Meaning of Suffering," *Sunstone* 18, no. 3 (1995): 37–43.

7. Ivan Illich, *Medical Nemesis: The Expropriation of Health* (New York: Pantheon, 1976); Peter Conrad, "Medicalization, Genetics and Human Problems," in *Handbook of Medical Sociology, 5th Edition*, ed. Chloe E. Bird, Peter Conrad, and Allen M. Fremont (Upper Saddle River: Prentice Hall, 2000), 322–33.

8. Cited in Daniel Callahan, *False Hopes: Why America's Quest for Perfect Health is a Recipe for Failure* (New York: Simon and Schuster, 1998), 30.

9. Campbell, "Ordeal and Meaning of Suffering," 37.

10. Stanley Hauerwas, *Suffering Presence: Theological Reflections on Medicine, the Mentally Handicapped, and the Church* (Notre Dame: University of Notre Dame Press, 1986), 24.

11. Campbell, "Ordeal and Meaning of Suffering," 37.

12. Smith, "Suffering, Medicine, and Christian Theology," 257.

13. Ibid., 259–60.

14. Ibid., 260.

15. Ibid., 257–58.

16. David M. Feldman, *Health and Medicine in the Jewish Tradition* (New York: Crossroad, 1986).

17. J. David Bleich, "The Obligation to Heal in the Judaic Tradition: A Comparative Analysis," in *Jewish Bioethics*, ed. Fred Rosner and J. David Bleich (New York: Sanhedrin Press, 1979), 17.

18. The survey asks the following: "In general, do you agree or disagree with the following statements: suffering is part of what makes us human." Those with the medical discourse of suffering should disagree with this: "1" is "strongly agree" and "4" is "strongly disagree." The correlation coefficient between the overall RGT index described in chap. 2 (higher numbers mean more opposition) and this variable is $-.134$ ($p < .001$). That is, those who believe that suffering has meaning in that it is part of what makes us human are more opposed to RGTs.

19. Details removed to protect anonymity.

20. Brackets in this quotation obscure details in order to protect anonymity.

21. See endnotes 11 and 12 in chap. 3 for a description of how pro-lifers and non–pro-lifers, as well as opponents and proponents, were demarcated using the survey.

22. The survey shows that conservative Protestants and Catholics are more likely than the nonreligious to claim that suffering has meaning. The effect is strongest for evangelicals, whereas mainline and liberal Protestants are no different from the secular respondents. I ran an ordered logistic regression model with the four-response meaningful suffering question (described above) as the dependent variable, where lower numbers indicate more agreement with the discourse, and dummy variables representing high attenders in the various religious traditions as the independent variables. Low attenders are the reference group. All coefficients significant at the $p < .05$ level except the mainline and liberal Protestant coefficients. The coefficients are as follows: Fundamentalist Protestant, $-.561$; Evangelical Protestant, $-.757$; Mainline Protestant, $-.179$; Liberal Protestant, $.016$; Traditionalist Catholic, $-.450$; Moderate Catholic, $-.325$; Liberal Catholic, $-.434$; and Other Attender, $-.373$.

23. Bill McKibben, "The Christian Paradox: How a Faithful Nation Gets Jesus Wrong," *Harpers* 311, no. 1863 (August 2005): 31.

Chapter Seven

1. Max Weber, *From Max Weber: Essays in Sociology*, trans. H. H. Gerth and C. Wright Mills (New York: Oxford University Press, 1946), 123.

2. Hunter, *Culture Wars* (New York: Basic Books, 1991), 42–51.

3. Ibid., 131.

4. This insight was, for many decades, the basis of secularization theory. Peter Berger, the modern synthesizer of this theory in sociology, argued that secular-

ization resulted from modern communications and travel ability, where for the first time in history it was easy for people with distinct worldviews to interact with each other. This interaction made both parties question the ultimate truth of their worldviews, resulting in a lack of certitude, which led to the weakening of religious faith in general. See Berger, *The Sacred Canopy: Elements of a Sociological Theory of Religion* (New York: Doubleday, 1967).

5. Cynthia B. Cohen, "Religious Belief, Politics, and Public Bioethics," *Second Opinion* 6 (2001): 37.

6. Gary S. Belkin, "Moving Beyond Bioethics: History and the Search for Medical Humanism," *Perspectives in Biology and Medicine* 47, no. 3 (2004): 375.

7. Robert Audi, "Liberal Democracy and the Place of Religion in Politics," in *Religion in the Public Square*, ed. Robert Audi and Nicholas Wolterstorff (Lanham: Rowman and Littlefield, 1997), 16. Or, as John Rawls, the father of modern discussions of political liberalism, writes, "Justification in matters of political justice is addressed to others who disagree with us, and therefore it proceeds from some consensus; from premises that we and others recognize as true, or as reasonable for the purpose of reaching a working agreement on the fundamentals of political justice." See John Rawls, "The Idea of Overlapping Consensus," *Oxford Journal of Legal Studies* 7, no. 1 (1987): 6.

8. John Rawls, *Political Liberalism* (New York: Columbia University Press, 1993).

9. Jean Bethke Elshtain, "Faith of Our Fathers and Mothers: Religious Belief and American Democracy," in *Religion in American Public Life*, ed. Azizah Y. al-Hibri, Jean Bethke Elshtain and Charles C. Haynes (New York: W. W. Norton, 2001), 39.

10. Alan Cooperman, "Openly Religious, to a Point: Bush Leaves the Specifics of His Faith to Speculation," *Washington Post* (Washington, DC), September 16, 2004, A:1.

11. Ibid.

12. President Delivers "State of the Union," (http://www.whitehouse.gov/news/releases/2003/01/20030128-19.html; accessed September 30, 2004).

13. The *Christian Century* further points out that the logic of this argument is that no religious motivations are allowed in the public sphere: "Try substituting 'infanticide' or 'slavery' for 'stem cell research', as in 'those who believe infanticide is wrong are entitled to their belief, but their theology should not forestall the well-being of the large society or the movement of history toward enlightenment." See "Stem Cell Rhetoric," *Christian Century* (Chicago), September 7, 2004, 5.

14. Robert Wuthnow and Conrad Hackett, "The Social Integration of Practitioners of Non-Western Religions in the United States," *Journal for the Scientific Study of Religion* 42, no. 4 (2003): 651–67.

15. Richard Madsen and Tracy B. Strong, "Introduction: Three Forms of Ethical Pluralism," in *The Many and the One*, ed. Richard Madsen and Tracy B. Strong (Princeton: Princeton University Press, 2003), 2.

16. Cherie Blair, "It is not just democracy that is illegal in Iran," *The Times*, July 9, 2009.

17. Paul Johnson, *A History of Christianity* (New York: Atheneum, 1976), 306.

18. Madsen and Strong, "Introduction: Three Forms of Ethical Pluralism," 3.

19. The ones that have not—arguably old-order Amish, Mennonites, some Orthodox Jews, and some Protestant fundamentalists—have intentionally marginalized themselves from public life.

20. Thomas Luckmann, *The Invisible Religion: The Problem of Religion in Modern Society* (New York: Macmillan, 1967).

21. José Casanova, *Public Religions in the Modern World* (Chicago: University of Chicago Press, 1994), 215.

22. The remainder volunteered responses such as "same as now" and "don't know." These data are from the "religion and politics" survey. For details about the survey, see Wuthnow and Evans, *The Quiet Hand of God: Faith-Based Activism and the Public Role of Mainline Protestantism*. The data are available at http://www.thearda.com. The survey was conducted between January 6 and March 31, 2000.

23. Mark D. Regnerus and Christian Smith, "Selective Deprivatization Among American Religious Traditions: The Reversal of the Great Reversal," *Social Forces* 76, no. 4 (1998): 1357. Regnerus and Smith found that the following percentages of respondents wanted religion to be involved in public life: attending fundamentalists (62.5 percent), attending evangelicals (68.3 percent), attending mainline Protestants (48.3 percent), attending liberal Protestants (37.3 percent), attending "other" Protestants (55.4 percent), "nominal" Protestants (26.5 percent), attending Catholics (34.5 percent), "nominal" Catholics (11.8 percent), non-Christians (23.3 percent), and nonreligious (15.5 percent).

24. "GOP the religion-friendly party," Report of the Pew Research Center for the people and the Press and the Pew Forum on Religion and Public Life, August 24, 2004, (http://people-press.org/reports/pdf/223.pdf).

25. The reference to the Hindu neighbor is made to evaluate the respondents' reaction to religious diversity by asking about someone who does not share any "lowest common denominator" Judeo-Christian beliefs.

26. The academic debate about the role of religion in public life has occurred almost exclusively on a theoretical level. There is an empirical literature that examines how religion-based social movement activists interact, but few studies of what the public thinks of this activism. See Christian Smith, *The Emergence of Liberation Theology: Radical Religion and Social-Movement Activism* (Chicago: University of Chicago Press, 1991); Christian Smith, *Disruptive Religion: The Force of Faith in Social-Movement Activism* (New York: Routledge, 1996); Richard L. Wood, *Faith in Action: Religion, Race and Democratic Organizing in America* (Chicago: University of Chicago Press, 2002); Mark R. Warren, *Dry Bones Rattling: Community Building to Revitalize American Democracy* (Princeton: Princeton University Press, 2001); Paul Lichterman, *Elusive Togetherness: Religion in the Quest for Civic Renewal* (Princeton: Princeton University Press, 2005); and Stephen Hart, *Cul-*

tural Dilemmas of Progressive Politics: Styles of Engagement Among Grassroots Activists (Chicago: University of Chicago Press, 2001). There is almost no empirical work on the use of religious discourse among ordinary citizens having discussions in the public sphere. Sociologists have written volumes on religion and politics, such as what people with different religious beliefs believe about certain policies, but have not focused on *how* that religion would actually be expressed in a public debate. The one more in-depth study of which I am aware is an interview study of middle-class Americans by Alan Wolfe, who found that—to simplify his findings greatly—Americans believe in being civil to each other when it comes to religion and politics. They do not want to exclude people from debates because of their religion, are concerned with pushing their views on others, and reject the idea that their religion has all of the answers. See Alan Wolfe, *One Nation, After All* (New York: Viking, 1998), chap. 2.

27. Wolfe, *One Nation, After All*, 53.

28. An interesting argument, found primarily among Catholics, is that secular arguments should be used because their religion believes in universal moral languages. That these Catholics use natural law theory like this suggests that the distinction between secular and religious arguments is Protestant in origin. See Heclo, *Christianity and American Democracy* (Cambridge: Harvard University Press, 2007).

29. Ethics and Religions Liberty Commission, For Faith and Family Issues, "Sanctity of human life fact sheet—2004."

30. The Apostle's creed is as follows: "I believe in God, the Father almighty, creator of heaven and earth. I believe in Jesus Christ, God's only Son, our Lord, who was conceived by the Holy Spirit, born of the Virgin Mary, suffered under Pontius Pilate, was crucified, died, and was buried; he descended to the dead. On the third day he rose again; he ascended into heaven, he is seated at the right hand of the Father, and he will come again to judge the living and the dead. I believe in the Holy Spirit, the Holy Catholic Church, the communion of saints, the forgiveness of sins, the resurrection of the body, and the life everlasting. AMEN." The Nicene Creed begins: "We believe in one God, the Father, the Almighty, maker of heaven and earth, of all that is, seen and unseen."

31. Robin W. Lovin, "Social Contract or a Public Covenant?" in *Religion and American Public Life: Interpretations and Explorations*, ed. Robin W. Lovin (New York: Paulist Press, 1986), 132.

32. N. J. Demerath, "Cultural Victory and Organizational Defeat in the Paradoxical Decline of Liberal Protestantism," *Journal for the Scientific Study of Religion* 34, no. 4 (1995): 460.

33. Wuthnow and Evans, *Quiet Hand of God: Faith-Based Activism and the Public Role of Mainline Protestantism*.

34. For an argument that atheists are the most discriminated against "religious" group, see Penny Edgell, Joseph Gerteis, and Douglas Hartmann, "Atheists as "Other": Moral Boundaries and Cultural Membership in American Society,"

American Sociological Review 71 (2006): 211–34; and Susan Jacoby, *Freethinkers: A History of American Secularism* (New York: Metropolitan Books, 2004).

35. Joel Robbins, "Ritual Communication and Linguistic Ideology: A Reading and Partial Reformulation of Rappaport's Theory of Ritual," *Current Anthropology* 42, no. 5 (2001): 598. On sincerity as the linguistic ideology of modernity, also see Joel Robbins, "God is Nothing but Talk: Modernity, Language and Prayer in a Papua New Guinea Society," *American Anthropologist* 103, no. 4 (2001); and Webb Keane, "From Fetishism to Sincerity: On Agency, the Speaking Subject, and Their Historicity in the Context of Religious Conversion," *Comparative Studies in Society and History* 39 (1997): 674–93.

Chapter Eight

1. Nigel Hawkes, "Human-cow hybrid embryo planned," *Times OnLine*, November 7, 2006; and Scott LaFee, "Spare Womb: Will Artificial Wombs Mean the End of Pregnancy?" San Diego Union-Tribune, February 25, 2004 (http://signonsandiego.com).

2. Ronald Cole-Turner, "Religion and the Question of Human Germline Modification," in *Design and Destiny: Jewish and Christian Perspectives on Human Germline Modification*, ed. Ronald Cole-Turner (Cambridge: MIT Press, 2008), 1–27.

3. Nigel M. de S. Cameron and Amy Michelle DeBaets, "Germline Gene Modification and the Human Condition Before God," 98, 107.

4. Ibid., 113, 114.

5. For a review of the disease/enhancement distinction in debates about human genetic engineering, see John H. Evans and Cynthia E. Schairer, "Bioethics and Human Genetic Engineering." See also LeRoy Walters and Julie Gage Palmer, *The Ethics of Human Gene Therapy* (New York: Oxford University Press, 1997), 109–11; Eric T. Juengst, "Can Enhancement Be Distinguished from Prevention in Genetic Medicine," *Journal of Medicine and Philosophy* 22 (1997): 126; and Erik Parens, "Is Better Always Good? The Enhancement Project," 5.

6. Francis Fukuyama, *Our Posthuman Future: Consequences of the Biotechnology Revolution*, 211.

7. Clearly, if current technologies were applied to humans, this would not be true, because huge numbers of cloned embryos have to be created to find one that will develop into a baby. Dolly the sheep was, for example, the one embryo of many that worked. I was more interested in what the religious public would think if cloning were to become efficient enough to not destroy embryos.

8. Leon Kass, "The Wisdom of Repugnance," 20.

9. National Bioethics Advisory Commission, *Cloning Human Beings: Report and Recommendations of the National Bioethics Advisory Commission* (Rockville: National Bioethics Advisory Commission, 1997).

10. Gilbert Meilaender, "Begetting and Cloning," *First Things* (June/July 1997): 42–43.

11. Jean Bethke Elshtain, "To Clone or not to Clone," in *Clones and Clones: Facts and Fantasies About Human Cloning*, ed. Martha C. Nussbaum and Cass R. Sunstein (New York: W. W. Norton, 1998), 182.

12. One of the primary ways of thinking about who is human in the Jewish and Christian traditions is to ask, "Who is made in the image of God?" Denominations and theologians agree that a clone would be just as human as the rest of us, also being made in the image of God. This can also be expressed with the language of human dignity. As a publication of a Catholic think tank put it, "In the cloning of humans there is an affront to human dignity . . . Yet, in no way is the human dignity of that person [the one who results from cloning] diminished." National Bioethics Advisory Commission, *Cloning Human Beings: Report and Recommendations of the National Bioethics Advisory Commission*, 50.

13. I also asked whether "this cloned child would have a soul." In retrospect, the question of whether a clone had a soul presumed the existence of a religious discourse about souls to which the ordinary member of a religion would have access. It may be interesting for theologians to know that almost all the respondents were a bit befuddled at having to talk about souls. It also makes no sense for the secular people, so it was not asked of them. However, like the "just as human as everyone else" question, this question is useful as an indicator of whether the people we spoke with think that a clone has the same status as they do, because even if people cannot give a theology of soul creation, they all know that they have one, according to their tradition. People almost always answered the two questions in the same way, suggesting that they are both indicators of the idea that a clone would be just as human as everyone else.

14. John Heritage, *Garfinkel and Ethnomethodology* (New York: Policy Press, 1984).

15. For a list of possible methods, see Ronald Cole-Turner, "Religion and the Question of Human Germline Modification."

16. This book is, in the terms used in the framing literature, a study of the ideology of the public before any framing begins. See Pamela E. Oliver and Hank Johnston, "What a Good Idea! Ideologies and Frames in Social Movement Research." The use of particular discourses by the respondents probably also varies by whom the person is trying to convince. I cannot examine this empirically because I have no variation in audience in the data. In the current case, I have no doubt that different discourses are used if the people are speaking in a group of people whom they know share the same religious tradition compared to a group of people who are not from their tradition. To be even more specific in my claims, this book is then about what discourses people use when faced with a general member of the public of indeterminate religious background, as embodied in the interviewer. It is probably also about how someone would converse with someone assumed to be "a

professor"—and all the political and social orientations that would imply—because the respondents knew that I was a professor and that the research assistants were aspiring professors. Of course, these constraints will exist for all interview-based research projects in the social sciences.

A second concern about question wording in social science research projects is broadly named the question-order effect, where, for example, making the respondents think of African Americans in the first question of a survey changes how they would otherwise respond to a second question about the government providing food stamps, because people secretly think that most African Americans are poor and they do not want to help poor African Americans. While people who design surveys often reflect on these issues, researchers using in-depth interviews rarely do, but the issues are the same. To use the language I have employed in this book, using one discourse predisposes someone toward using it again, so if a respondent uses a discourse with the first question about abortion, they are more likely to use it than they otherwise would for the second question about preimplantation genetic diagnosis.

There is no technical fix for this problem and no ability to measure the size of a question-order effect outside of experimental surveys and social psychology laboratory experiments. The only solution is to be aware of the potential effect and to then limit the claims being made. The most conservative limitation of my claims would assume that there is a strong question order effect. Specifically, this would mean that the strong opponents use the four discourses I focused on to discuss abortion for cystic fibrosis, and only used those discourses for later questions because they used them for the first. Therefore, if I had not asked about abortion, they would have used different discourses. However, note that even this most conservative limitation of my claims fits with the most likely scenario for how opposition to RGTs will be introduced into the public sphere, which is by the antiabortion movement. People would then, in the future, have the same response I am showing here because, like a society-wide interview, the right to life movement would be cuing the abortion debate by linking opposition to the new RGTs to opposition to abortion. By this most conservative interpretation, this book would be most applicable if it is the antiabortion movement that promotes anti-RGT discourse in the public sphere.

However, the results presented in this book can also be interpreted to show that there is no consequential question-order effect. Most notably, the (relative) proponents, who are often pro-choice on abortion, talk about abortion early in the interview but do not use the three strongly oppositional discourses that I focus on in this book. Then, when the conversations get to enhancements, they do use these discourses, talking like the strong opponents. This suggests that the use of the discourses I focus on is not dependent on first using them in a discussion about abortion. So, this book can be interpreted as applicable to the full range of future situations.

17. James Hunter, *Culture Wars*; Hunter, *Before the Shooting Begins*; Paul DiMaggio, John Evans, and Bethany Bryson, "Have Americans' Social Attitudes

Become More Polarized?"; Evans, "Have Americans' Attitudes Become More Polarized?—an Update"; Fiorina, *Culture War? The Myth of a Polarized America.*

18. Keith T. Poole and Howard Rosenthal, "D-NOMINATE After 10 Years: A Comparative Update to Congress: A Political-Economic History of Roll-Call Voting," *Legislative Studies Quarterly* 26, no. 1 (2001): 5–29.

19. Philip E. Converse, "The Nature of Belief Systems in Mass Publics," in *Ideology and Discontent*, ed. David E. Apter (New York: Free Press, 1964), 206–61; M. Kent Jennings, "Ideological Thinking Among Mass Publics and Political Elites," *Public Opinion Quarterly* 56 (1992): 419–41; and Christopher M. Federico and Monica C. Schneider, "Political Expertise and the Use of Ideology: Moderating Effects of Evaluative Motivation," *Public Opinion Quarterly* 71, no. 2 (2007): 221–52.

20. See endnote 50, chap. 1.

21. Christopher M. Federico and Monica C. Schneider, "Political Expertise and the Use of Ideology: Moderating Effects of Evaluative Motivation," 223.

22. Hunter, *Before the Shooting Begins.*

23. Hunter, *Culture Wars.*

24. Ted G. Jelen and Clyde Wilcox, "Causes and Consequences of Public Attitudes Toward Abortion: A Review and Research Agenda," 498.

25. Social movement scholars call this "frame extension," whereas social problems scholars call it "domain expansion," both of which are extremely similar concepts. Generalizing across studies, two scholars conclude that expansion can lead to "murkiness" in argumentation because a new, broader discourse needs to be used for the new expanded domain. Debra Friedman and Doug McAdam, "Collective Identity and Activism: Networks, Choices and the Life of a Social Movement," in *Frontiers in Social Movement Theory*, ed. Aldon D. Morris and Carol McClurg Mueller (New Haven: Yale University Press, 1992), 164–65. Similarly, in a study of the case where the antiabortion group Operation Rescue tried to engage in domain expansion to include opposition to homosexuality and pornography, they had to turn to a discourse of reconstructionist theology. "For reconstructionists, all three of Operation Rescue's protest targets . . . represent the ongoing modernization and secularization of American society," writes sociologist Nicole Youngman. For the activists, these issues were all the same because they are all logically implied by "modernization and secularization." Youngman quotes an Operation Rescue leader talking to the press who says: "It's the same arena, you have to understand . . . We are dealing with two world views, a culture of death vs. a culture of life . . . the homosexual world view is exactly the same as the world view of abortion . . . "I'll do what I want whenever I want to, and the one commandment I have is 'thou shalt not get in my face, and don't you dare judge me!' " . . . It's not a battle about abortion or homosexuality, it's a battle about whose laws reign, or who is Lord, and we're saying that Jesus is Lord and Mickey is not." This discourse about a "modernist secularism" is incredibly abstract.

To put it simply, potential debating partners who are initially opposed to your perspective are not going to know what this incredibly abstract discourse means. Youngman concludes that one of the reasons Operation Rescue failed was because "their framing simply *made no sense* to anyone outside the religious right who was not already well-versed in Reconstructionist theology." Youngman, "When Frame Extension Fails: Operation Rescue and the 'Triple Gates of Hell' in Orlando," 529, 535.

26. See, e.g., Nina Eliasoph, *Avoiding Politics: How Americans Produce Apathy in Everyday Life* (New York: Cambridge University Press, 1998).

Appendix A

1. Egon Mayer, Barry Kosmin, and Ariela Keysar, "American Jewish Identity Survey 2001," Center for Jewish Studies, Graduate Center of the City University of New York, 2002.

2. It should be of no surprise that the primarily non-Jewish religious elites in our elite survey did not really know the difference between reform and reconstructionist Judaism, so the primary reform congregation in one of our cities ended up actually being reconstructionist. In my conversations with the Rabbi and my examination of their web pages I determined that this congregation would serve as a legitimate substitute. To massively over-simplify, reconstructionism can be thought of as a ritualistically more conservative than reform, yet theologically more liberal. There is obviously a huge range in belief and practice among reconstructionist and reform synagogues.

3. Wuthnow and Evans, *The Quiet Hand of God: Faith-Based Activism and the Public Role of Mainline Protestantism*, 4.

4. Ibid.

5. Mark Chaves, Helen M. Giesel, and William Tsitsos, "Religious Variations in Public Presence: Evidence from the National Congregations Study," in *The Quiet Hand of God: Faith-Based Activism and the Public Role of Mainline Protestantism*, ed. Robert Wuthnow and John H. Evans (Berkeley and Los Angeles: University of California Press, 2002), 114.

6. Ibid.

7. "New Study Reveals Hispanics at Center of Catholic Church in the United States" (http://www.nccbuscc.org/comm/archives/2000/00-044.shtml).

8. Chaves, Giesel, and Tsitsos, "Religious Variations in Public Presence: Evidence from the National Congregations Study," 114.

9. Sargeant, *Seeker Churches: Promoting Traditional Religion in a Nontraditional Way*; Miller, *Reinventing American Protestantism: Christianity in the New Millennium*.

10. Knowledge Networks has created a series of papers for reviewers that discuss method, representativeness and the construction of weights (see http://www.knowledgenetworks.com/ganp/reviewer-info.html).

11. That survey was the religion and politics survey, available at the Association of Religion Data Archives (http://www.thearda.com). The survey was conducted between January 6 and March 31, 2000. The Knowledge Networks survey had 2.1 percent more fundamentalists, 2.1 percent more evangelicals, 0.3 percent more mainline Protestants, 1.1 percent more liberal Protestants, 1.4 percent fewer traditional Catholics, 2.1 percent fewer moderate Catholics, and 0.3 percent more liberal Catholics. Of course, there is no way of telling which survey is a true measure of religious preference in the United States.

Works Cited

Ahlstrom, Sydney. 1972. *A religious history of the American people.* New Haven: Yale University Press.

Almond, Douglas, and Lena Edlund. 2008. Son-biased sex ratios in the 2000 United States Census. *Proceedings of the National Academy of Sciences* 105, no. 15: 5681–82.

Anderson, Rebecca Rae. 2002. *Religious traditions and prenatal genetic counseling.* Omaha: Munroe-Meyer Institute, University of Nebraska Medical Center.

Arnhart, Larry. 2003. Darwinian conservatism as the new natural law. *Good Society* 12, no. 3: 14–19.

Ashcroft, Richard E. 2005. Making sense of dignity. *Journal of Medical Ethics* 31:679–82.

Audi, Robert. 1997. Liberal democracy and the place of religion in politics. In *Religion in the Public Square.* Edited by Robert Audi and Nicholas Wolterstorff. Lanham: Rowman and Littlefield, 1–66.

Bane, Audra, Lesli Brown, Joy Carter, Chris Cote, Karin Crider, Suzanne de la Forest, Michelle Livingston, and Darrel Montero. 2003. Life and death decisions: America's changing attitudes toward genetic engineering, genetic testing and abortion, 1972–98. *International Social Work* 46, no. 2: 209–19.

Bates, Benjamin R., John A. Lynch, Jennifer L. Bevan, and Celeste M. Condit. 2005. Warranted concerns, warranted outlooks: A focus group study of public understandings of genetic research. *Social Science and Medicine* 60:331–44.

Becker, Gay. 2000. *The elusive embryo: How women and men approach new reproductive technologies.* Berkeley and Los Angeles: University of California Press.

Belkin, Gary S. 2004. Moving beyond bioethics: History and the search for medical humanism. *Perspectives in Biology and Medicine* 47, no. 3: 372–85.

Berger, Peter L. 1967. *The sacred canopy: Elements of a sociological theory of religion.* New York: Doubleday.

———. 1999. The desecularization of the world: A global overview. In *The desecularization of the world: Resurgent religion and world politics.* Edited by Peter L. Berger. Grand Rapids: Eerdmans, 1 18.

Best, Joel. 1990. *Threatened children: Rhetoric and concern about child-victims.* Chicago: University of Chicago Press.

———. 1999. *Random violence: How we talk about new crimes and new victims.* Berkeley and Los Angeles: University of California Press.

———. 2008. *Social problems.* New York: W. W. Norton.

Bleich, J. David. 1979. The obligation to heal in the Judaic tradition: A comparative analysis. In *Jewish bioethics.* Edited by Fred Rosner and J. David Bleich. New York: Sanhedrin Press, 1–44.

Bleiklie, Ivar, Malcolm L. Goggin, and Christine Rothmayr. 2004. *Comparative biomedical policy: Governing assisted reproductive technologies.* London and New York: Routledge.

Boeyink, David E. 1974. Pain and suffering. *Journal of Religious Ethics* 2:85–98.

Boyle, James. 1998. How to give natures a chance. *Times Literary Supplement,* July 24, 21–22.

Bulger, Ruth Ellen, Elizabeth Meyer Bobby, and Harvey V. Fineberg. 1995. *Society's choices: Social and ethical decision making in biomedicine.* Washington, DC: National Academy Press.

Callahan, Daniel. 1998. *False hopes: Why America's quest for perfect health is a recipe for failure.* New York: Simon and Schuster.

Campbell, Courtney S. 1995. "The ordeal and meaning of suffering." *Sunstone* 18, no. 3: 37–43.

Caplan, Arthur. 2005. "'Who lost China?' A foreshadowing of today's ideological disputes in bioethics." *Hastings Center Report* 35, no. 3: 12–13.

Carmen, Arlene, and Howard Moody. 1973. *Abortion counseling and social change from illegal act to medical practice: The story of the clergy consultation service on abortion.* Valley Forge: Judson Press.

Casanova, José. 1994. *Public religions in the modern world.* Chicago: University of Chicago Press.

Cassell, Eric J. 1991. *The nature of suffering and the goals of medicine.* New York: Oxford University Press.

Caulfield, Timothy, and Roger Brownsword. 2006. Human dignity: A guide to policy making in the biotechnology era? *Nature Reviews Genetics* 7:72–76.

Cerulo, Karen A. 2002. *Culture in mind: Toward a sociology of culture and cognition.* New York: Routledge.

Chaves, Mark, Helen M. Giesel, and William Tsitsos. 2002. Religious variations in public presence: Evidence from the National Congregations Study. In *The quiet hand of God: Faith-based activism and the public role of mainline Protestantism.* Edited by Robert Wuthnow and John H. Evans. Berkeley and Los Angeles: University of California Press, 108–28.

Christian Century. 2004. Stem cell rhetoric. *Christian Century* (Chicago, IL), September 7, 5.

Cohen, Cynthia B. 2001. Religious belief, politics, and public bioethics. *Second Opinion* 6:37–52.

Cohen, Eric. 2003. Of embryos and empire. *The New Atlantis* 2:3–16.

Cole-Turner, Ronald. 2008. Religion and the question of human germline modification. In *Design and destiny: Jewish and Christian perspectives on human germline modification*. Edited by Ronald Cole-Turner. Cambridge: MIT Press, 1–27.

Condit, Celeste M. 1999. How the public understands genetics: Non-deterministic and non-discriminatory interpretations of the "blueprint" metaphor. *Public Understanding of Science* 8:169–80.

Conrad, Peter. 2000. Medicalization, genetics and human problems. In *Handbook of medical sociology, 5th edition*. Edited by Chloe E. Bird, Peter Conrad, and Allen M. Fremont. Upper Saddle River: Prentice Hall, 322–33.

Converse, Philip E. 1964. The nature of belief systems in mass publics. In *Ideology and discontent*. Edited by David E. Apter. New York: Free Press, 206–61.

Cooperman, Alan. 2004. Openly religious, to a point: Bush leaves the specifics of his faith to speculation. *Washington Post*, September 16, A:1.

Daston, Lorraine, and Fernando Vidal. 2004. *The moral authority of nature*. Chicago: University of Chicago Press.

Davis, Joseph E. 2005. *Accounts of innocence: Sexual abuse, trauma, and the self.* Chicago: University of Chicago Press.

Davis, Nancy J., and Robert V. Robinson. 1996. Are rumors of war exaggerated? Religious orthodoxy and moral progressivism in America. *American Journal of Sociology* 102, no. 3 (November): 756–76.

Davis, Tom. 2005. *Sacred work: Planned Parenthood and its clergy alliances*. New Brunswick: Rutgers University Press.

de S. Cameron, Nigel M., and Amy Michelle DeBaets. 2008. Germline gene modification and the human condition before God. In *Design and destiny: Jewish and Christian perspectives on human germline modification*. Edited by Ronald Cole-Turner. Cambridge: MIT Press, 93–118.

Delli Carpini, Michael X., Fay Lomax Cook, and Lawrence R. Jacobs. 2004. Public deliberation, discursive participation, and citizen engagement: A review of the empirical literature. *Annual Review of Political Science* 7:315–44.

Demerath, N. J. 1995. Cultural victory and organizational defeat in the paradoxical decline of liberal Protestantism. *Journal for the Scientific Study of Religion* 34, no. 4: 458–69.

Dillon, Michele. 1993. Argumentative complexity of abortion discourse. *Public Opinion Quarterly* 57:305–14.

———. 1995. Institutional legitimation and abortion: Monitoring the Catholic Church's discourse. *Journal for the Scientific Study of Religion* 34, no. 2: 141–51.

———. 1996. The American abortion debate: Culture war or normal discourse? In *The American culture wars: Current contests and future prospects*. Edited by James L. Nolan. Charlottesville: University Press of Virginia, 115–32.

DiMaggio, Paul. 1997. Culture and cognition. *Annual Review of Sociology* 23: 263–87.

DiMaggio, Paul, John Evans, and Bethany Bryson. 1996. Have Americans' social attitudes become more polarized? *American Journal of Sociology* 102:690–755.

DiMaggio, Paul, and Walter W. Powell. 1991. Introduction. In *The new institutionalism in organizational analysis*. Edited by Walter W. Powell and Paul J. DiMaggio. Chicago: University of Chicago Press, 1–40.

Douglas, Mary. 1986. *How institutions think*. Syracuse: Syracuse University Press.

Durkheim, Emile. 1951. *Suicide.* New York: Free Press.

Duster, Troy. 1990. *Backdoor to eugenics.* New York: Routledge.

Ecklund, Elaine Howard. 2010. *Science vs. religion: What do scientists really think?* New York: Oxford University Press.

Ecklund, Elaine Howard, and Christopher P. Scheitle. 2007. Religion among academic scientists: Distinctions, disciplines, and demographics. *Social Problems* 54, no. 2: 289–307.

Edgell, Penny, Joseph Gerteis, and Douglas Hartmann. 2006. Atheists as "other": Moral boundaries and cultural membership in American Society. *American Sociological Review* 71:211–34.

Edwards, R.G., and Ruth E. Fowler. 1970. Human embryos in the laboratory. *Scientific American* 223, no. 6: 44–54.

Eliasoph, Nina. 1998. *Avoiding politics: How Americans produce apathy in everyday life.* New York: Cambridge University Press.

Eliasoph, Nina, and Paul Lichterman. 2003. Culture in interaction. *American Journal of Sociology* 108, no. 4: 735–94.

Elshtain, Jean Bethke. 1998. To clone or not to clone. In *Clones and clones: Facts and fantasies about human cloning.* Edited by Martha C. Nussbaum and Cass R. Sunstein. New York: W. W. Norton, 181–89.

———. 2001. Faith of our fathers and mothers: Religious belief and American democracy. In *Religion in American public life.* Edited by Azizah Y. al-Hibri, Jean Bethke Elshtain, and Charles C. Haynes. New York: W. W. Norton, 39–61.

Emerson, Michael O., and Christian Smith. 2000. *Divided by faith: Evangelical religion and the problem of race.* New York: Oxford University Press.

Ettorre, Elizabeth. 2002. *Reproductive genetics, gender and the body.* London and New York: Routledge.

Evans, John H. 1997. Multi-organizational fields and social movement organization frame content: The religious pro-choice movement. *Sociological Inquiry* 67, no. 4: 451–69.

———. 1997. Worldviews or social groups as the source of moral value attitudes: Implications for the culture wars thesis. *Sociological Forum* 12, no. 3: 371–404.

———. 2002. *Playing God? Human genetic engineering and the rationalization of public bioethical debate.* Chicago: University of Chicago Press.

———. 2002. Polarization in abortion attitudes in U.S. religious traditions 1972–1998. *Sociological Forum* 17, no. 3: 397–422.

———. 2002. Religion and human cloning: An exploratory analysis of the first available opinion data. *Journal for the Scientific Study of Religion* 41, no. 4: 747–58.

———. 2003. Have Americans' attitudes become more polarized?—An update. *Social Science Quarterly* 84, no. 1: 71–90.

———. 2006. Between technocracy and democratic legitimation: A proposed compromise position for common morality public bioethics. *Journal of Medicine and Philosophy* 31: 213–34.

———. 2006. Religious belief, perceptions of human suffering and support for reproductive genetic technology. *Journal of Health Politics, Policy and Law* 31, no. 6: 1047–74.

Evans, John H., and Kathy Hudson. 2007. Religion and reproductive genetics: Beyond views of embryonic life? *Journal for the Scientific Study of Religion* 46, no. 4: 565–81.

Evans, John H., and Cynthia E. Schairer. 2009. Bioethics and human genetic engineering. In *Handbook of genetics and society: Mapping the new genomic era.* Edited by Paul Atkinson, Peter Glasner, and Margaret Lock. London: Routledge, 349–66.

Federico, Christopher M., and Monica C. Schneider. 2007. Political expertise and the use of ideology: Moderating effects of evaluative motivation. *Public Opinion Quarterly* 71, no. 2: 221–52.

Feldman, David M. 1986. *Health and medicine in the Jewish tradition.* New York: Crossroad.

Ferree, Myra Marx, William A. Gamson, Jurgen Gerhards, and Dieter Rucht. 2002. *Shaping abortion discourse: Democracy and the public sphere in Germany and the United States.* Cambridge and New York: Cambridge University Press.

Fiorina, Morris. 2005. *Culture war? The myth of a polarized America.* New York: Pearson Longman.

Fiske, Susan T., and Shelley E. Taylor. 1991. *Social cognition.* New York: McGraw-Hill.

Fletcher, John. 1972. The Brink: The parent-child bond in the genetic revolution. *Theological Studies* 33, no. 3: 457–85.

Fletcher, Joseph. 1971. Ethical aspects of genetic controls. *New England Journal of Medicine* 285, no. 14: 776–83.

Franklin, Monica D., David G. Schlundt, and Kenneth A. Wallston. 2008. Development and validation of a religious health fatalism measure for the African American faith community. *Journal of Health Psychology* 13, no. 3: 323–35.

Franklin, Sarah. 1997. *Embodied Progress: A Cultural Account of Assisted Conception.* London and New York: Routledge.

Friedman, Debra, and Doug McAdam. 1992. Collective identity and activism: Networks, choices and the life of a social movement. In *Frontiers in social movement theory.* Edited by Aldon D. Morris and Carol McClurg Mueller. New Haven: Yale University Press, 156–73.

Frum, David. 2008. The vanishing Republican voter: Why income inequality is destroying the G.O.P. base. *New York Times* (Sunday Magazine), September 7, 48–51.

Fukuyama, Francis. 2002. *Our posthuman future: Consequences of the biotechnology revolution.* New York: Farrar, Straus and Giroux.

Garrow, David J. 1994. *Liberty and sexuality: The right to privacy and the making of Roe v. Wade.* New York: Macmillan/Lisa Drew.

Gelernter, David. 2008. The irreducibly religious character of human dignity. In *Human Dignity and Bioethics,* 387–405. Washington, DC: President's Council on Bioethics.

Genetics and Public Policy Center. 2004. Reproductive Genetic Testing: Issues and Options for Policymakers, Washington, DC.

Gerring, John. 1997. Ideology: A definitional analysis. *Political Research Quarterly* 50, no. 4: 957–94.

Glass, Bentley. 1965. *Science and ethical values.* Chapel Hill: University of North Carolina Press.

Goi, Simona. 2005. Agonism, deliberation and the politics of abortion. *Polity* 37, no. 1: 54–81.

Greeley, Andrew. 1989. Protestant and Catholic: Is the analogical imagination extinct? *American Sociological Review* 54:485–502.

———. 2000. *The Catholic imagination.* Berkeley and Los Angeles: University of California Press.

Gross, Neil, and Solon Simmons. 2009. The religiosity of American college and university professors. *Sociology of Religion* 70: 101–29.

Gutmann, Amy, and Dennis Thompson. 1996. *Democracy and disagreement.* Cambridge: Harvard University Press.

Haldane, John H. 2003. Natural law and ethical pluralism. In *The many and the one.* Edited by Richard Madsen and Tracy B. Strong. Princeton: Princeton University Press, 89–114.

Hall, Amy Laura. 2008. *Conceiving parenthood: American Protestantism and the spirit of reproduction.* Grand Rapids: Eerdmans.

Handyside, A. H., E. H. Kontogianni, K. Hardy, and R. M. L. Winston. 1990. Pregnancies from biopsied human preimplantation embryos sexed by Y-specific DNA amplification. *Nature* 344:768–70.

Harris, John. 1998. *Clones, genes and immortality: Ethics and the genetic revolution.* New York: Oxford University Press.

———. 2007. *Enhancing Evolution: The ethical case for making better people.* Princeton: Princeton University Press.

Hart, Stephen. 2001. *Cultural dilemmas of progressive politics: Styles of engagement among grassroots activists.* Chicago: University of Chicago Press.

Hauerwas, Stanley. 1986. *Suffering resence: Theological reflections on medicine, the mentally handicapped, and the Church.* Notre Dame: University of Notre Dame Press.

Heclo, Hugh. 2007. *Christianity and American democracy.* Cambridge: Harvard University Press.

Henderson, Mark. 2004. Gene tests to start era of baby-to-order. *The Times* (London), June 26, 1.

Henneman, L., I. Bramsen, Th. A. M. Van Os, I. E. W. Reuling, H. G. M. Heyerman, J. van der Laag, H. M. van der Ploeg, and L. P. ten Kate. 2001. Attitudes toward reproductive issues and carrier testing among adult patients and parents of children with cystic fibrosis (CF). *Prenatal Diagnosis* 21:1–9.

Heritage, John. 1984. *Garfinkel and ethnomethodology.* New York: Polity Press.

Hopkins, Patrick D. 2002. Protecting God from science and technology: How religious criticisms of biotechnologies backfire. *Zygon* 37, no. 2: 317–43.

Huckfeldt, Robert. 2007. Unanimity, discord, and the communication of public opinion. *American Journal of Political Science* 51, no. 4: 978–95.

Hulse, Carl. 2009. Democrats weigh methods for ending stem cell ban. *New York Times,* January 3, A:11.

Hunter, James D. 1991. *Culture wars.* New York: Basic Books.

———. 1994. *Before the shooting begins.* New York: Free Press.

Hunter, James. 1983. *American evangelicalism: Conservative religion and the quandary of modernity.* New Brunswick: Rutgers University Press.

Huxley, Julian. 1963. Eugenics in evolutionary perspective. *Perspectives in Biology and Medicine* (Winter): 155–87.

Illich, Ivan. 1976. *Medical nemesis: The expropriation of health.* New York: Pantheon.

Iredale, Rachel, Marcus Longley, Christian Thomas, and Anita Shaw. 2006. What choices should we be able to make about designer babies? A citizens' jury of young people in South Wales. *Health Expectations* 9:207–17.

Jacoby, Susan. 2004. *Freethinkers: A history of American secularism.* New York: Metropolitan Books.

Jelen, Ted G., and Clyde Wilcox. 2003. Causes and consequences of public attitudes toward abortion: A review and research agenda. *Political Research Quarterly* 56, no. 4: 489–500.

Jenness, Valerie. 1995. Social movement growth, domain expansion, and framing processes: The gay/lesbian movement and violence against gays and lesbians as a social problem. *Social Problems* 42, no. 1: 145–70.

Jennings, M. Kent. 1992. Ideological thinking among mass publics and political elites. *Public Opinion Quarterly* 56:419–41.

Johnson, Paul. 1976. *A history of Christianity.* New York: Atheneum.

Juengst, Eric T. 1997. Can enhancement be distinguished from prevention in genetic medicine. *Journal of Medicine and Philosophy* 22:125–42.

Kalfoglou, Andrea L., Teresa Doksum, Barbara Bernhardt, Gail Geller, Lisa Le-Roy, Debra Mathews, John H. Evans, David J. Doukas, Nancy Ream, Joan Scott, and Kathy Hudson. 2005. Opinions about new reproductive genetic technologies: Hopes and fears for our genetic future. *Fertility and Sterility* 83, no. 6: 1612–21.

Kass, Leon R. 1997. The wisdom of repugnance. *New Republic,* June 2, 17–26.

———. 2008. Defending human dignity. In *Human Dignity and Bioethics,* 297–332. Washington, DC: President's Council on Bioethics.

Keane, Webb. 1997. From fetishism to sincerity: On agency, the speaking subject, and their historicity in the context of religious conversion. *Comparative Studies in Society and History* 39:674–93.

Kevles, Daniel. 1985. *In the name of eugenics: Genetics and the uses of human heredity.* Berkeley and Los Angeles: University of California Press.

Keys, Mary M. 1995. Personal dignity and the common good: A twentieth-century Thomistic dialogue. In *Catholicism, liberalism, and communitarianism: The Catholic intellectual tradition and the moral foundations of democracy.* Edited by Kenneth L. Grasso, Gerard V. Bradley, and Robert P. Hunt. Lanham: Rowman and Littlefield, 173–96.

Learman, Lee A., Miriam Kuppermann, Elena Gates, Robert F. Nease, Virginia Gildengorin, and A. Eugene Washington. 2003. Social and familial context of prenatal genetic testing decisions: Are there racial/ethnic differences. *American Journal of Medical Genetics Part C* 119:19–26.

Lee, Thomas F. 1991. *The Human Genome Project: Cracking the genetic code of life.* New York: Plenum Press.

Lichterman, Paul. 2005. *Elusive togetherness: Religion in the quest for civic renewal.* Princeton: Princeton University Press.

Liebman, Robert C., and Robert Wuthnow, eds. 1983. *The New Christian Right.* New York: Aldine.

Loseke, Donileen R. 1999. *Thinking about social problems: An introduction to constructionist perspectives.* New York: Aldine de Gruyter.

Lovin, Robin W. 1986. Social contract or a public covenant? In *Religion and American public life: Interpretations and explorations.* Edited by Robin W. Lovin. New York: Paulist Press, 132–45.

Luckmann, Thomas. 1967. *The invisible religion: The problem of religion in modern society.* New York: Macmillan.

Luker, Kristin. 1984. *Abortion and the politics of motherhood.* Berkeley and Los Angeles: University of California Press.

Macklin, Ruth. 2003. Dignity is a useless concept. *BMJ* 327:1419–20.

Madsen, Richard, and Tracy B. Strong. 2003. Introduction: Three forms of ethical pluralism. In *The many and the one.* Edited by Richard Madsen and Tracy B. Strong. Princeton: Princeton University Press, 1–21.

Mayer, Egon, Barry Kosmin, and Ariela Keysar. 2002. American Jewish identity survey 2001. Center for Jewish Studies, Graduate Center of the City University of New York.

McKibben, Bill. 2005. The Christian paradox: How a faithful nation gets Jesus wrong. *Harpers* 311, no. 1863 (August): 31–37.

Meagher, Richard J. 2006. Tax revolt as a family value: How the Christian right is becoming a freemarket champion. *Public Eye Magazine* 21, no. 1.

Meilaender, Gilbert. 1997. Begetting and cloning. *First Things* (June/July): 41–43.

———. 2001. Designing our descendants. *First Things* 109 (January): 25–28.

Melton, J. Gordon. 1989. *The churches speak on: Abortion.* Detroit: Gale Research.

Miller, Donald E. 1997. *Reinventing American Protestantism: Christianity in the new millennium.* Berkeley and Los Angeles: University of California Press.

Mohr, James C. 1978. *Abortion in America: The origins and evolution of national policy.* New York: Oxford University Press.

Moon, Dawne. 2004. *God, sex and politics: Homosexuality and everyday theologies.* Chicago: University of Chicago Press.

Muller, Hermann J. 1959. The guidance of human evolution. *Perspectives in Biology and Medicine* 3, no. 1: 1–43.

———. 1965. Means and aims in human betterment. In *The control of human heredity and evolution.* Edited by T. M. Sonneborn. New York: Macmillan, 100–22.

Mutz, Diana C. 2002. Cross-cutting social networks: Testing democratic theory in practice. *American Political Science Review* 96, no. 1: 111–26.

———. 2008. Is deliberative democracy a falsifiable theory? *Annual Review of Political Science* 11:521–38.

Mutz, Diana C., and Paul S. Martin. 2001. Facilitating communication across lines of political difference: The role of the mass media. *American Political Science Review* 95, no. 1: 97–114.

Naik, Gautam. 2009. A baby, please. Blond, freckles—hold the colic. *Wall Street Journal Online,* February 12.

National Bioethics Advisory Commission. 1997. *Cloning human beings: Report and recommendations of the National Bioethics Advisory Commission.* Rockville: National Bioethics Advisory Commission.

Nisbet, Robert. 1994. *History of the idea of progress.* New Brunswick: Transaction Press.

Oliver, Pamela E., and Hank Johnston. 2000. What a good idea! Ideologies and frames in social movement research. *Mobilization* 4, no. 1: 37–54.

Parens, Erik. 1998. Is better always good? The enhancement project. In *Enhancing human traits: Ethical and social implications.* Edited by Erik Parens. Washington, DC: Georgetown University Press, 1–28.

Parens, Erik, and Lori P. Knowles. 2003. Reprogenetics and public policy: Reflections and recommendations. *Hastings Center Report* 33, no. 4: S1–S24.

Paul, Diane B. 1995. *Controlling human heredity: 1865 to the present.* Amherst: Humanity Books.

Peffley, Mark A., and Jon Hurwitz. 1985. A hierarchical model of attitude constraint. *American Journal of Political Science* 29:871–89.

Pence, Gregory E. 1998. *Who's afraid of human cloning?* Lanham: Rowman and Littlefield.

Perrin, Andrew J. 2005. Political microcultures: Linking civic life and democratic discourse. *Social Forces* 84, no. 2.

Peters, Ted. 2003. *Playing God? Genetic determinism and human freedom.* New York: Routledge.

Poole, Keith T., and Howard Rosenthal. 2001. D-NOMINATE after 10 years: A comparative update to Congress: A political-economic history of roll-call voting. *Legislative Studies Quarterly* 26, no. 1: 5–29.

President's Council on Bioethics. 2002. *Human cloning and human dignity: An ethical inquiry.* Washington, DC: President's Council on Bioethics.

———. 2003. *Beyond therapy: Biotechnology and the pursuit of happiness.* Washington, DC: President's Council on Bioethics.

———. 2008. *Human dignity and bioethics.* Washington, DC: President's Council on Bioethics.

Pullman, Daryl. 2001. Universalism, particularism and the ethics of dignity. *Christian Bioethics* 7, no. 3: 333–58.

Ramsey, Paul. 1970. *Fabricated man: The ethics of genetic control.* New Haven: Yale University Press.

Rapp, Rayna. 1999. *Testing women, testing the fetus: The social impact of amniocentesis in America.* New York: Routledge.

Rawls, John. 1987. The idea of overlapping consensus. *Oxford Journal of Legal Studies* 7, no. 1: 1–25.

———. 1993. *Political Liberalism.* New York: Columbia University Press.

Regnerus, Mark D., and Christian Smith. 1998. Selective deprivatization among American religious traditions: The reversal of the great reversal. *Social Forces* 76, no. 4: 1347–72.

Reich, Warren Thomas. 1989. Speaking of suffering: A moral account of compassion. *Soundings* 72, no. 1: 83–108.

Reichhardt, Tony. 2004. Studies of faith. *Nature* 432:666–69.

Robbins, Joel. 2001. God is nothing but talk: Modernity, language and prayer in a Papua New Guinea society. *American Anthropologist* 103, no. 4.

———. 2001. Ritual communication and linguistic ideology: A reading and partial reformulation of Rappaport's theory of ritual. *Current Anthropology* 42, no. 5: 591–99.

Rorvik, David M. 1978. *In His image: The cloning of a man.* Philadelphia: Lippincott.

Rosen, Christine. 2004. *Preaching eugenics: Religious leaders and the American eugenics movement.* New York: Oxford University Press.

Rothman, Barbara Katz. 1986. *The tentative pregnancy: Prenatal diagnosis and the future of motherhood.* New York: Viking.

———. 1989. *Recreating motherhood: Ideology and technology in a patriarchal society.* New York: Norton.

Ryfe, David M. 2002. The practice of deliberative democracy: A study of sixteen organizations. *Political Communication* 16:359–78.

———. 2005. Does deliberative democracy work? *Annual Review of Political Science* 8: 49–71.

Sargeant, Kimon Howland. 2000. *Seeker churches: Promoting traditional religion in a nontraditional way.* New Brunswick: Rutgers University Press.

Sewell, Jr., William H. 1999. The concept(s) of culture. In *Beyond the cultural turn: New directions in the study of society and culture.* Edited by Victoria E. Bonnell and Lynn Hunt. Berkeley and Los Angeles: University of California Press, 35–61.

Shepherd, Richard, Julie Bernett, Helen Cooper, Adrian Coyle, Jo Moran-Ellis, Victoria Senior, and Chris Walton. 2007. Towards an understanding of British public attitudes concerning human cloning. *Social Science and Medicine* 65:377–92.

Silber, Ilana Friedrich. 2003. Pragmatic sociology as cultural sociology: Beyond repertoire theory? *European Journal of Social Theory* 6, no. 4: 427–49.

Silver, Lee M. 2000. Reprogenetics: How reproductive and genetic technologies will be combined to provide new opportunities for people to reach their reproductive goals. In *Engineering the Human Germline.* Edited by Gregory Stock and John Campbell. New York: Oxford University Press, 57–71.

Singer, Eleanor. 1991. Public attitudes toward genetic testing. *Population Research and Policy Review* 10: 235–55.

Singer, Eleanor, Toni Antonucci, and John Van Hoewyk. 2004. Racial and ethnic variations in knowledge and attitudes about genetic testing. *Genetic Testing* 8, no. 1: 31–43.

Singer, Eleanor, Amy D. Corning, and Toni Antonucci. 1999. Attitudes toward genetic testing and fetal diagnosis. *Journal of Health and Social Behavior* 40:429–45.

Singer, Eleanor, Amy Corning, and Mark Lamias. 1998. The polls—trends: Genetic testing, engineering and therapy. *Public Opinion Quarterly* 62:633–64.

Smith, Christian. 1991. *The emergence of liberation theology: Radical religion and social-movement activism.* Chicago: University of Chicago Press.

————. 1996. *Disruptive religion: The force of faith in social-movement activism.* New York: Routledge.

————. 1998. *American evangelicalism: Embattled and thriving.* Chicago: University of Chicago Press.

Smith, David H. 1987. Suffering, medicine, and Christian theology. In *On moral medicine: Theological perspectives in medical ethics.* Edited by Stephen E. Lammers and Allen Verhey. Grand Rapids: Eerdmans, 255–61.

Snow, David A., and Robert D. Benford. 1992. Master frames and cycles of protest. In *Frontiers in social movement theory.* Edited by Aldon D. Morris and Carol McClurg Mueller. New Haven: Yale University Press, 133–55.

Snow, David A., E. Burke Rochford, Jr., Steven K. Worden, and Robert D. Benford. 1986. Frame alignment processes, micromobilization, and movement participation. *American Sociological Review* 51:464–81.

Sonneborn, Tracy M. 1965. *The control of human heredity and evolution.* New York: Macmillan.

Soper, Kate. 1995. *What is Nature? Culture, politics, and the non-human.* Cambridge: Blackwell.

Steensland, Brian, Jerry Z. Park, Mark D. Regnerus, Lynn D. Robinson, W. Bradford Wilcox, and Robert D. Woodberry. 2000. The measure of American religion: Toward improving the state of the art. *Social Forces* 79, no. 1: 291–318.

Strickler, Jennifer, and Nicholas L. Danigelis. 2002. Changing frameworks in attitudes toward abortion. *Sociological Forum* 17, no. 2: 187–201.

Swanson, Guy E. 1967. *Religion and regime: A sociological account of the Reformation.* Ann Arbor: University of Michigan Press.

Swidler, Ann. 1986. Culture in action: Symbols and strategies. *American Sociological Review* 51: 273–86.

————. 2001. *Talk of love: How culture matters.* Chicago: University of Chicago Press.

Taylor, Charles. 1995. Liberal politics and the public sphere. In *The new communitarian thinking.* Edited by Amitai Etzioni. Charlottesville: University Press of Virginia, 183–217.

Thuesen, Peter J. 2002. The logic of mainline churchliness: Historical background since the Reformation. In *The quiet hand of God: Faith-based activism and the public role of mainline Protestantism.* Edited by Robert Wuthnow and John H. Evans. Berkeley and Los Angeles: University of California Press, 27–53.

Tribe, Laurence. 1992. *Abortion: The clash of absolutes.* New York: Norton.

Verhey, Allen. 1995. "Playing God" and invoking a perspective. *Journal of Medicine and Philosophy* 20:347–64.

Verlinsky, Y., S. Rechitsky, O. Verlinsky, C. Masciangelo, K. Lederer, and A. Kuliev. 2002. Preimplantation diagnosis for early-onset Alzheimer disease caused by V717L mutation. *JAMA* 287, no. 8: 1018–21.

Walters, LeRoy, and Julie Gage Palmer. 1997. *The ethics of human gene therapy.* New York: Oxford University Press.

Warren, Mark R. 2001. *Dry bones rattling: Community building to revitalize American democracy.* Princeton: Princeton University Press.

Weber, Max. 1946. *From Max Weber: Essays in sociology.* Translated by H. H. Gerth and C. Wright Mills. New York: Oxford University Press.

Wertz, Dorothy C., and John C. Fletcher. 2004. *Genetics and ethics in global perspective.* Dordrecht: Kluwer Academic.

Wertz, Dorothy, S. R. Janes, and R. W. Erbe. 1992. Attitudes toward the prenatal diagnosis of cystic fibrosis factors in decision-making among affected families. *American Journal of Human Genetics* 50, no. 5: 1077–85.

Witten, Marsha. 1993. *All is forgiven: The secular message in American Protestantism.* Princeton: Princeton University Press.

Wolfe, Alan. 1998. *One nation, after all.* New York: Viking.

Wood, Richard L. 2002. *Faith in action: Religion, race and Democratic organizing in America.* Chicago: University of Chicago Press.

Woodberry, Robert D., and Christian S. Smith. 1998. Fundamentalism et al: Conservative Protestants in America. *Annual Review of Sociology* 24:25–56.

Wuthnow, Robert, and John H. Evans, eds. 2002. *The quiet hand of God: Faith-based activism and the public role of mainline Protestantism.* Berkeley and Los Angeles: University of California Press.

Wuthnow, Robert, and Conrad Hackett. 2003. The social integration of practitioners of non-Western religions in the United States. *Journal for the Scientific Study of Religion* 42, no. 4: 651–67.

Yang, Yonghe, and N. J. Demerath III. 1997. What American culture war? A view from the trenches as opposed to the command posts and the press corps. In *Cultural Wars in American Politics: Critical Reviews of a Popular Thesis.* Edited by Rhys H. Williams. Hawthorn: Aldine de Gruyter.

Youngman, Nicole. 2003. When frame extension fails: Operation Rescue and the "triple gates of hell" in Orlando. *Journal of Contemporary Ethnography* 32, no. 5: 521–54.

Index